Bowel Ultrasound Compared with Endoscopy

Springer Nature More Media App

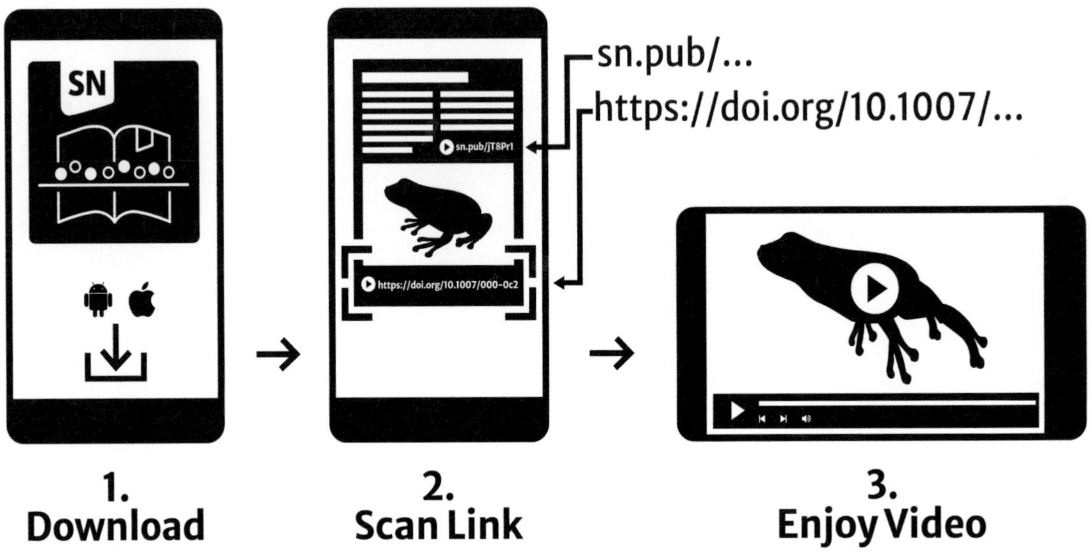

Support: customerservice@springernature.com

Fulvia Terracciano • Antonella Marra
Fabrizio Bossa
Editors

Bowel Ultrasound Compared with Endoscopy

Springer

Editors
Fulvia Terracciano
Division of Gastroenterology and Digestive Endoscopy
Fondazione IRCCS "Casa Sollievo della Sofferenza"
San Giovanni Rotondo, Italy

Antonella Marra
National Institute of Gastroenterology
IRCCS "Saverio de Bellis" Research Hospital
Castellana Grotte, Italy

Fabrizio Bossa
Division of Gastroenterology and Digestive Endoscopy
Fondazione IRCCS "Casa Sollievo della Sofferenza"
San Giovanni Rotondo, Italy

This work contains media enhancements, which are displayed with a "play" icon. Material in the print book can be viewed on a mobile device by downloading the Springer Nature "More Media" app available in the major app stores. The media enhancements in the online version of the work can be accessed directly by authorized users.

ISBN 978-3-032-11417-4 ISBN 978-3-032-11418-1 (eBook)
https://doi.org/10.1007/978-3-032-11418-1

This Springer imprint is published by the registered company Springer Nature Switzerland AG
The registered company address is: Gewerbestrasse 11, 6330 Cham, Switzerland

Foreword

In an era dominated by digital technology, where knowledge is increasingly accessed through screens, the printed pages of a book might seem like a relic of the past—belonging to a time when human understanding took shape in texts that remained unaltered over time and space. And yet, holding this book in hand and leafing through its pages, enriched with remarkable and carefully curated iconography, one immediately appreciates the power of the printed format. The clarity and depth conveyed through paper and high-quality images enhance the learning experience in a way that digital formats often struggle to match.

This book is the result of a shared passion among its authors—many of whom are pioneers in the field of gastrointestinal ultrasound. Once considered a complex and niche technique, reserved for only a handful of experts, intestinal ultrasound has since gained widespread recognition for its clinical utility. This manual and atlas represents one of the few, if not the only, dedicated resources available for those engaged in this evolving discipline. By presenting its subject matter with clarity and accessibility, it helps demystify the "*shadows*" created by ultrasound waves as they interact with the human body.

The book has been expertly compiled by three esteemed colleagues, Fulvia, Antonella, and Fabrizio, whom I had the privilege of working with during my professional activity at the Casa Sollievo della Sofferenza Hospital in San Giovanni Rotondo. It brings together the contributions of leading specialists, with a particular focus on the area where intestinal ultrasound has had its most significant clinical impact: chronic inflammatory bowel diseases (IBD), including ulcerative colitis and Crohn's disease.

With the global prevalence of IBD rising, these conditions represent a growing challenge for specialists, particularly in diagnosis, disease activity monitoring, and the detection of complications during treatment. In this regard, intestinal ultrasound has emerged as a fundamental tool, offering a cost-effective, safe, and widely available imaging technique that has revolutionized patient care.

Beyond its current applications, intestinal ultrasound is also opening new frontiers in IBD management. The development of IUS-based predictive models and AI-driven diagnostic tools holds the promise of transforming clinical decision-making, enabling early therapeutic interventions, tight-control monitoring, and, ultimately, improved disease outcomes.

While this book is an invaluable resource for IBD specialists, its reach extends far beyond. It serves as a reference for all professionals in the field of imaging diagnostics, particularly those who frequently encounter patients with gastrointestinal disorders that are newly presenting or difficult to interpret.

It is my hope that this work will establish itself as a key reference in the international scientific literature and an essential learning tool for those embarking on their journey into this dynamic and evolving field.

Head of the Department of Gastroenterology
and Digestive Endoscopy Diseases
IRCCS Casa Sollievo della Sofferenza
San Giovanni Rotondo, Foggia, Italy

Francesco Perri

Preface

Ultrasound is a discipline of remarkable beauty. From the very beginning of my work, it captured my attention with its extraordinary ability to reveal the complexity of the human body. My passion for this technology was born out of curiosity and a desire to explore, but it was also supported by the immense dedication, wisdom, and kindness of two exceptional mentors: Ilario De Sio and Luigi Castellano. They taught me that ultrasound is far more than a diagnostic tool: it is a privileged window into the human body.

Over the years, thanks Prof. Angelo Andriulli, farsighted and brilliant primary, my enthusiasm for ultrasound has continued to grow, driven not only by the discovery of the technique's potential but also by a profound desire to share this knowledge. Teaching has become an essential part of my professional life, based on the belief that passing on my expertise to future generations is one of the most challenging endeavors.

Writing this atlas has been both a journey of discovery and the realization of a long-held dream. It represents not only the culmination of years of experience but also my unwavering commitment to education. Teaching, for me, is not merely the transmission of knowledge—it is a shared experience that enriches both teacher and student. Every lesson, every interaction, and every exchange of ideas has strengthened my conviction that education is a cornerstone of professional growth and personal fulfillment.

The completion of this project, like any dream brought to fruition, would not have been possible without the support of those who believed in me and contributed to its success. I am deeply grateful to everyone who accompanied me along this journey, each playing a unique role in bringing this atlas to life. To my husband, whose unwavering support and encouragement made everything possible. To Luigi and Antonio, my sons, who bore the sacrifices of my absence. I hope they have learned that in giving, one often receives much more in return. To my family, my safe and ever-present refuge, my harbor. To Fabrizio, one of the most knowledgeable, humble, and precise professionals I know, and a constant reference point in the field of inflammatory bowel diseases. To Chiara, Leonardo, and Veronica, my team, whose lively intelligence always made everything seem light and joyful. To Antonella, who worked on this dream more than anyone else, making it her own. Her determination, intelligence, and remarkable professionalism have far exceeded my highest expectations. Watching her grow into an extraordinary clinician and person has been one of the greatest privileges of my career. Without her, this work would not exist.

Finally, I dedicate this atlas to all those who will embark on the fascinating journey of ultrasound, with their hands on the transducer and their minds and hearts open to discovery. My hope is that this book will serve as a guide and source of inspiration, illuminating the extraordinary beauty and potential of every ultrasound image.

San Giovanni Rotondo, FG, Italy Fulvia Terracciano

Acknowledgment

We are grateful to the Italian Group for the Study of Inflammatory Bowel Disease (IG-IBD) and the International Bowel Ultrasound Group (IBUS Group) for their sponsorship and support. Both organizations are dedicated to promoting worldwide knowledge of intestinal ultrasound, which is the focus of this work.

Contents

About the Editors

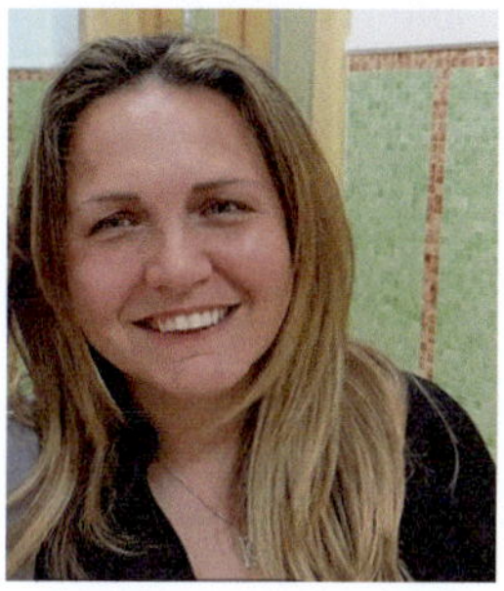

Fulvia Terracciano has been in the Division of Gastroenterology and Endoscopy at the IRCSS Casa Sollievo della Sofferenza in San Giovanni Rotondo, ITALY, since 2007. She specializes in diagnostic and interventional abdominal ultrasound and has extensive experience in hepatology and inflammatory bowel diseases, as well as in performing abdominal, transperineal, intestinal ultrasounds, and ultrasound-guided interventional procedures. She is a member and lecturer of the IBUS Group (International Bowel Ultrasound), SIUMB (Italian Society of Medical and Biological Ultrasound), and IG-IBD (Italian Group for Inflammatory Bowel Disease). She is also a speaker at numerous national and international ultrasound congresses. She is a Coordinator and Lecturer at the SIUMB Advanced School of Gastroenterology, the IG-IBD Master Program, and the IBUS Center of San Giovanni Rotondo. She is co-author of several publications on abdominal and intestinal ultrasound. She currently serves as a principal and sub-investigator in many studies on inflammatory bowel diseases.

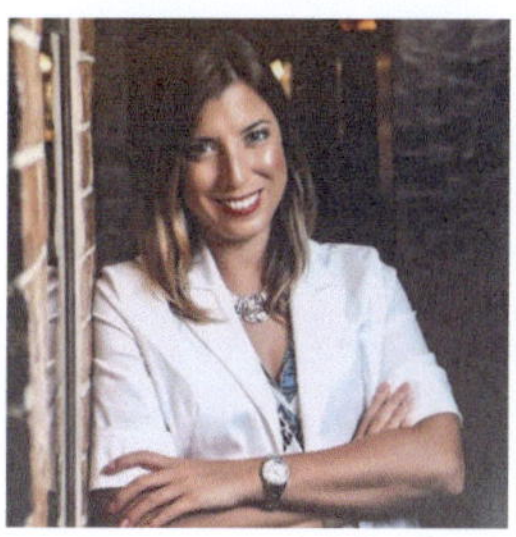

Antonella Marra was born in 1988 and graduated in Medicine from the University of Florence. She subsequently completed her specialization in Gastroenterology in Bari and obtained a Master's degree in diagnostic and interventional ultrasound at the University of Foggia. She currently works at the National Institute of Gastroenterology, IRCCS "S. De Bellis", in Castellana Grotte, Italy. She has always focused her clinical and research activity on ultrasound, developing particular expertise in bowel ultrasound, and she has participated as a sub-investigator in several clinical studies on IBD. She also works as a tutor at the Basic Ultrasound School and the Advanced School of

Gastroenterology. She is a member of the IBUS Group (International Bowel Ultrasound), SIUMB (Italian Society of Medical and Biological Ultrasound), and IG-IBD (Italian Group for Inflammatory Bowel Disease).

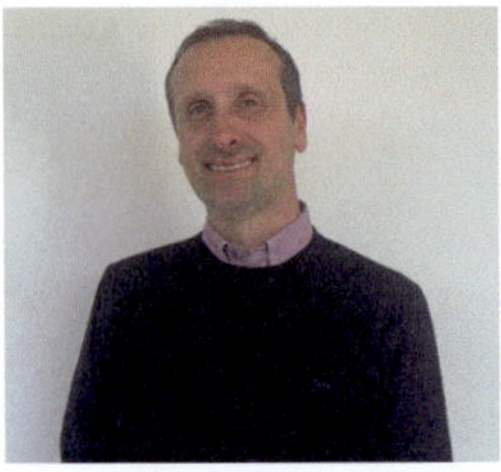

Fabrizio Bossa was born in 1973 and graduated in Medicine at the University of Naples, specializing in Gastroenterology. Since 2005 he has been working at the Gastroenterology Department of the Casa Sollievo della Sofferenza Hospital in San Giovanni Rotondo where his main interest is inflammatory bowel diseases (IBD). He works as a tutor in the Basic Ultrasound School and the IBUS International Ultrasound School.

Normal Gastrointestinal Tracts 1

Antonella Marra, Paola Dell'Aquila,
Veronica Nassisi, and Fulvia Terracciano

1.1 Introduction

For many years, the gastrointestinal tract was considered as unsuitable for ultrasound examination due to the presence of gas-related artifacts. However, studies from the 1970s first highlighted the potential utility of this technique for bowel assessment [1, 2]. Recently, technological advancements have largely overcome the obstacles associated with using ultrasound for evaluating different gastrointestinal diseases.

Supplementary Information The online version contains supplementary material available at https://doi.org/10.1007/978-3-032-11418-1_1. The videos can be accessed individually by clicking the DOI link in the accompanying figure caption or by scanning this link with the SN More Media App.

A. Marra (✉)
National Institute of Gastroenterology,
IRCCS "Saverio de Bellis" Research Hospital,
Castellana Grotte, Italy
e-mail: antonella.marra@irccsdebellis.it

P. Dell'Aquila
Section of Gastroenterology, Department
of Emergency and Organ Transplantation,
University of Bari, Bari, Italy

V. Nassisi
General Medicine Unit, "Casa di Cura San Camillo",
Messina, Italy

F. Terracciano
Division of Gastroenterology and Digestive
Endoscopy, Fondazione IRCCS "Casa Sollievo della
Sofferenza", San Giovanni Rotondo, Italy

1.2 Execution Technique and Basic Principles

Gaseous content within the intestine, due to its high acoustic impedance, results in total reflection of the ultrasound beam. The presence of air alone, or in combination with liquid and/or solid contents, generates gas-related artifacts, including horizontal reverberations, ring-down artifacts, and posterior acoustic shadowing, allowing visualization of the anterior bowel wall only (Fig. 1.1). As gaseous content decreases, whether due to physiological (e.g., ingestion of food or water) or pathological conditions (e.g., wall thickening, malabsorption) a real image is obtained, without artifacts, with visualization of both the anterior and posterior walls (Fig. 1.2).

The ultrasound examination is performed with the patient in a supine position, after fasting for at least 6–8 hours, and with a moderately distended bladder. It is not recommended for patients to drink water before the examination, as this may lead to misdiagnosis of malabsorption disorders or cause bladder overdistension, which could displace the small bowel.

A low-frequency convex (3.5–5 MHz) probe is initially employed for a panoramic assessment, followed by a high-frequency linear probe

F. Terracciano et al. (eds.), *Bowel Ultrasound Compared with Endoscopy*,
https://doi.org/10.1007/978-3-032-11418-1_1

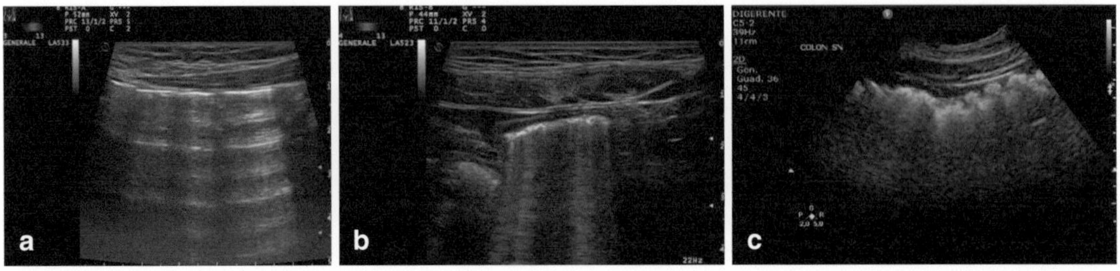

Fig. 1.1 (**a**) Horizontal reverberation artifact, predominantly gaseous content; (**b**) Vertical reverberation or ring-down artifact, mixed intraluminal content (fluid + gas); (**c**) 'Dirty' acoustic shadowing, mixed luminal content with a predominant solid component. In all three images, only the anterior bowel wall is visible, while the posterior wall is obscured by the artifact

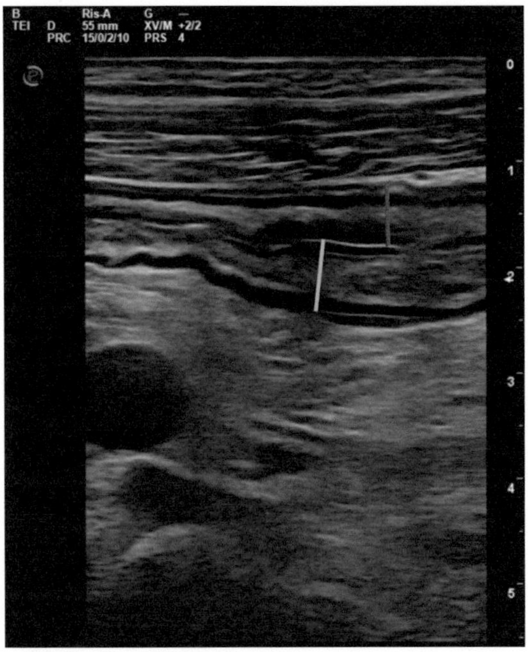

Fig. 1.2 Thickened ileal segment in a patient with Crohn's disease. Both anterior (red line) and posterior (green line) bowel walls are clearly identified

(4–13 MHz) to provide detailed visualization. Longitudinal, transverse, and oblique scans are utilized as appropriate for the specific segment under examination [3].

1.3 Normal Sonographic Features

The main features of the bowel wall evaluated by ultrasound include wall thickness, echogenic pattern, vascularity, and motility. Among these, echogenicity and wall thickening represent the most important features in identifying gastrointestinal diseases. The frequency of the probe and the pressure applied by the operator can significantly affect the ultrasound appearance of the gastrointestinal tract. Given its tubular structure, the bowel generally displays a 'target' sign in transverse scans and as a 'track' in longitudinal scans (Fig. 1.3).

1.3.1 Bowel Wall Pattern and Thickness

The normal bowel wall is stratified into five distinct layers with different echogenicity. Starting from the luminal side, the first is the interface between the lumen (hyperechoic) and the mucosa (hypoechoic); the remaining layers include: submucosa (hyperechoic), muscularis propria (hypoechoic), and serosa (hyperechoic). Wall thickness is the main ultrasonographic feature of

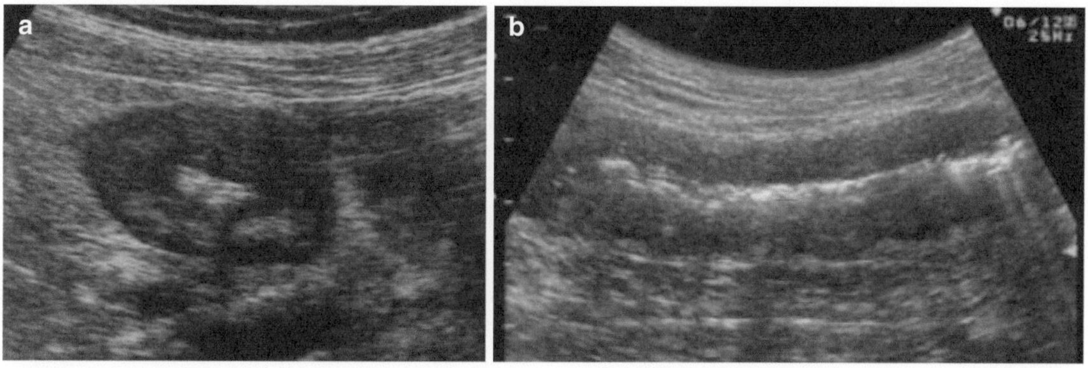

Fig. 1.3 Gut displays a 'target' sign in transverse scan (**a**) and as a 'track' in longitudinal scan (**b**)

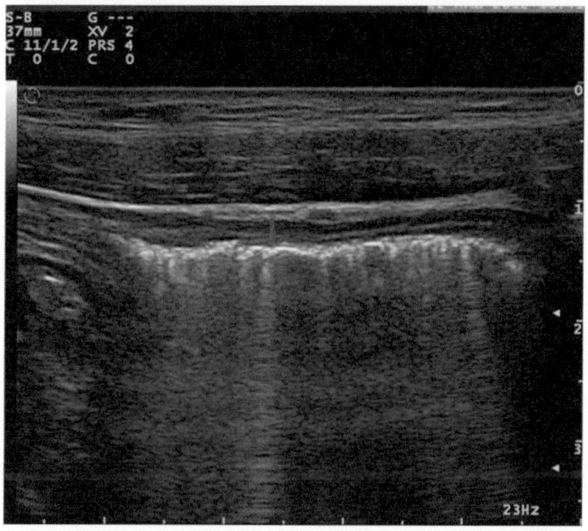

Fig. 1.4 Measurements of bowel wall thickening should be taken from the external hyperechoic layer to the internal hyperechoic layer, perpendicular to the axis of the lumen, at the point of greatest thickening, preferentially in the anterior wall, avoiding haustration and mucosal folds (red line)

the gut assessed by ultrasound. Measurements of bowel wall thickening should be taken using a high frequency probe, from the external hyperechoic layer (serosa) to the internal hyperechoic layer (interface between mucosa and lumen), perpendicular to the axis of the lumen, at the point of greatest thickening, preferentially in the anterior wall, avoiding haustration and mucosal folds (Fig. 1.4). The stomach wall thickness ranges between 2 and 7 mm [4]; the small bowel has a thickness up to 3 mm; while the colon, particularly in the sigmoid, has a normal thickness of up to 5 mm [5].

1.3.2 Luminal Content

Normal luminal content may be absent or gaseous, liquid, solid, or mixed. An empty intestine displays collapsed walls, with a thin hyperechoic line (mucosa-luminal interface) between the visible anterior and posterior walls. When the content is gaseous, reverberation artifacts (such as 'ring down') can obscure the posterior wall, allowing visualization of the anterior wall only. Gradual compression of the bowel can displace the gas, enabling better visualization of the posterior wall. Liquid content appears anechoic, allowing visualization of both the anterior and posterior walls, with the internal mucosal profile typically well-defined (Fig. 1.5). When liquids are mixed with solid or gaseous components, they present as a corpuscular medium. The ultrasound image shows spots of varying sizes and echogenicity. The solid component may appear as a stone-like structure with posterior acoustic shadowing. This type of content is generally observed in the colon, especially in constipated patients (Fig. 1.6) [6].

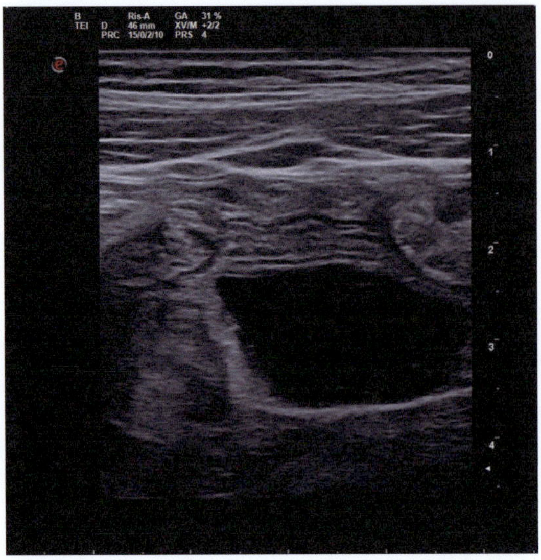

Fig. 1.5 Small bowel containing fluid (anechoic) is observed in transverse scan, allowing clear delineation of the mucosal profile as well as the anterior and posterior bowel walls

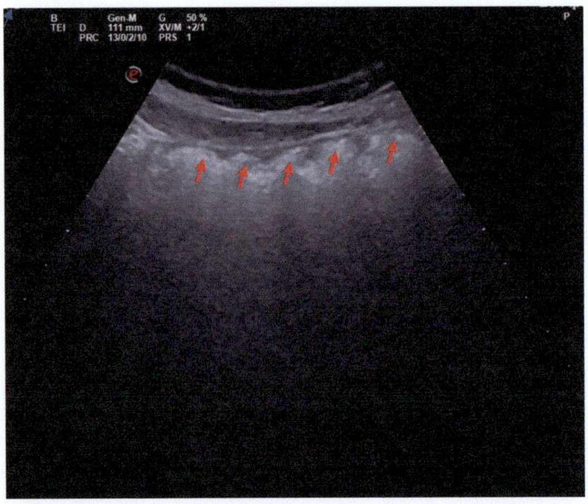

Fig. 1.6 Colon with enteric content predominantly solid, producing dirty acoustic shadowing. Colonic haustrations are clearly visualized (arrows)

1.4 Normal Gastrointestinal Tract

1.4.1 Esophagus

The cervical esophagus can be examined by scanning the left side of the midline of the neck using a linear probe, through both transverse and longitudinal scans. It is located 2–3 cm from the skin surface, posterior to the left thyroid lobe, laterally to the trachea. In transverse scans, it appears circular and target-like, while in longitudinal scans, it appears tubular. Typically, its lumen is collapsed but becomes visible when a salivary bolus passes through (Fig. 1.7).

The thoracic esophagus cannot be assessed with transthoracic ultrasound due to the presence of the rib cage, but it can be examined using endoscopic ultrasound (EUS).

The terminal esophagus is sub-diaphragmatic and can be visualized through longitudinal and transverse epigastric scans to the left of the caudate lobe using a convex probe. The terminal esophagus and the esophagogastric junction are anterior to the aorta and posterior to the caudate lobe (Fig. 1.8).

1.4.2 Stomach

The gastric wall thickness ranges from 2 to 7 mm, depending on its functional status (contraction or relaxation). To improve visualization of the gastric walls, the intake of 500 mL of water before the examination is recommended. The visibility of the body-fundic region is often limited due to its deep location within the abdomen and the presence of air; it can be visualized through left

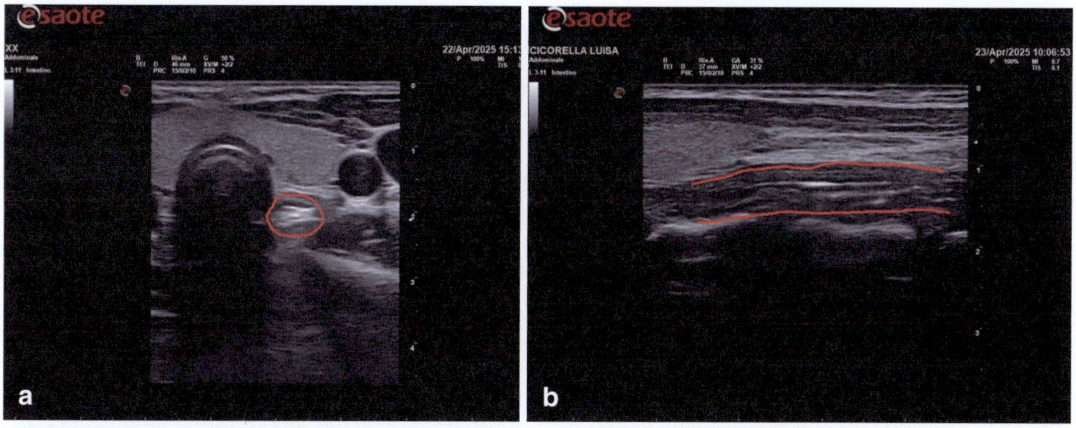

Fig. 1.7 Transverse (**a**) and longitudinal (**b**) sonographic sections of the cervical esophagus (red line)

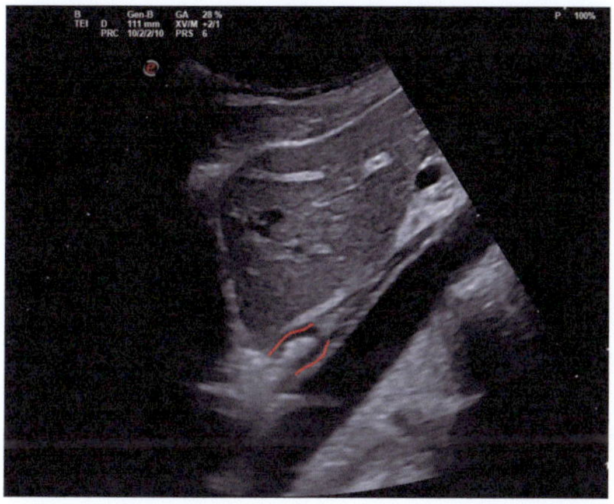

Fig. 1.8 The terminal esophagus and the gastroesophageal junction are located anterior to the aorta and posterior to the left liver lobe (red lines)

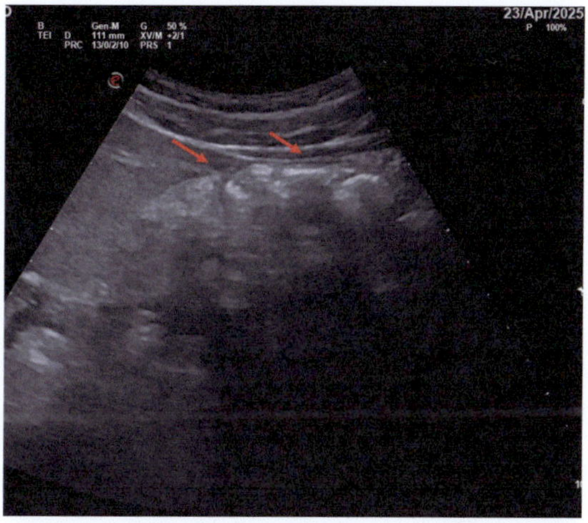

Fig. 1.9 Left subcostal ascending scan: gastric body containing predominantly air (arrows)

subcostal ascending scans (Fig. 1.9) or left-sided intercostal coronal scans (Fig. 1.10). It is placed medial to the left hepatic lobe, anterior to the tail of the pancreas, and lateral to the spleen.

The antral-pyloric region is well visualized because it is more superficial. It is placed posterior to the left hepatic lobe and anterior to the body of the pancreas (Fig. 1.11).

1.4.3 Duodenum

The duodenum is divided into four parts: duodenal bulb, descending, horizontal, and ascending portions. The duodenal bulb appears as a tubular

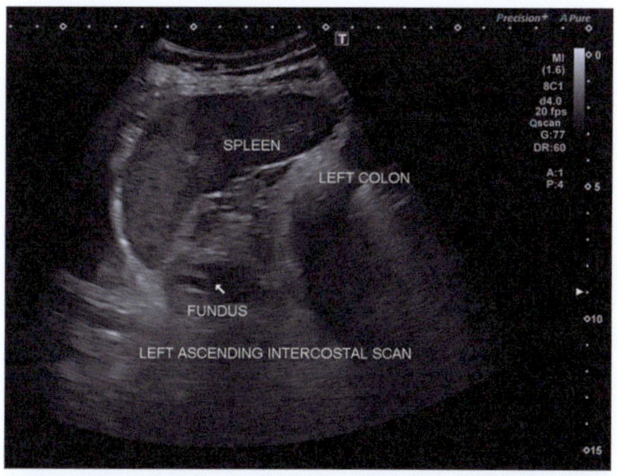

Fig. 1.10 Left ascending intercostal scan: the gastric fundus is visualized near the upper pole of the spleen

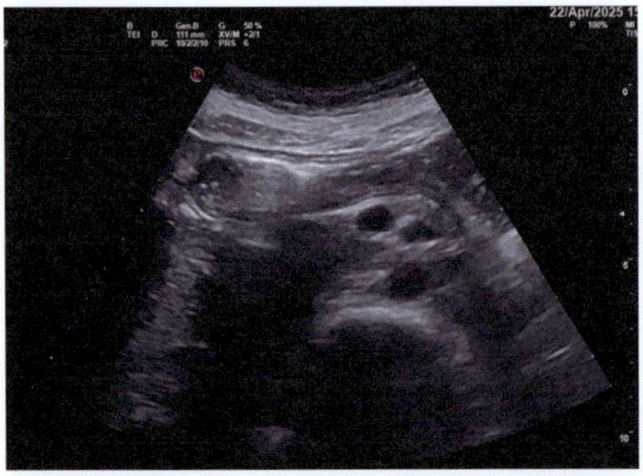

Fig. 1.11 Transverse scan in the epigastric region: the antral-pyloric region is visualized

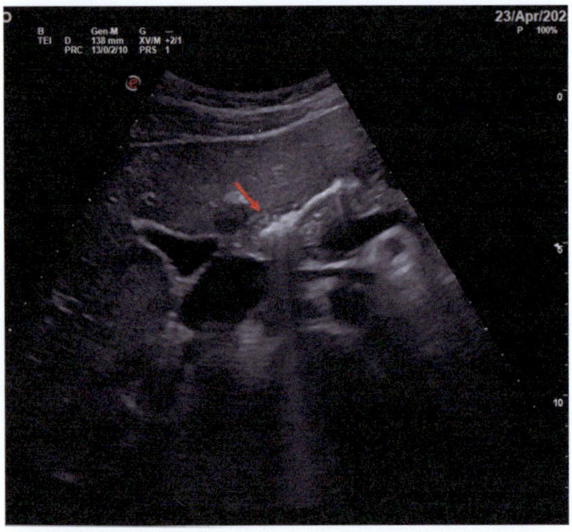

Fig. 1.12 Duodenal bulb containing air (arrow)

structure containing mainly gas. It is located posterior to the left hepatic lobe, medial to the gallbladder infundibulum and anterior to the head of the pancreas (Fig. 1.12). The descending duodenum, or the second portion, is located anteromedial to the right kidney, lateral to the inferior vena cava, and posterior to the gallbladder. When filled with fluid, duodenal folds are visible as small, finger-like extensions within the lumen (Fig. 1.13).

The third portion of the duodenum is visualized with axial scans in the epi-mesogastrium and it is located between the superior mesenteric artery and the aorta. Often, it is difficult to assess due to its deep positioning, the interposition of the transverse colon and collapsed lumen (Fig. 1.14).

The ascending portion is positioned posterior to the stomach, and often the gas contained in the fundus and body of the stomach prevents its visualization.

1.4.4 Small Bowel

The small bowel is the most challenging segment of the gastrointestinal tract to explore due to the lack of anatomical landmarks. Therefore, abdominal quadrants are used to identify the anatomical location of potential pathological changes. The only two segments that have landmarks are the jejunum immediately distal to the ligament of Treitz and the terminal ileum. The study of the

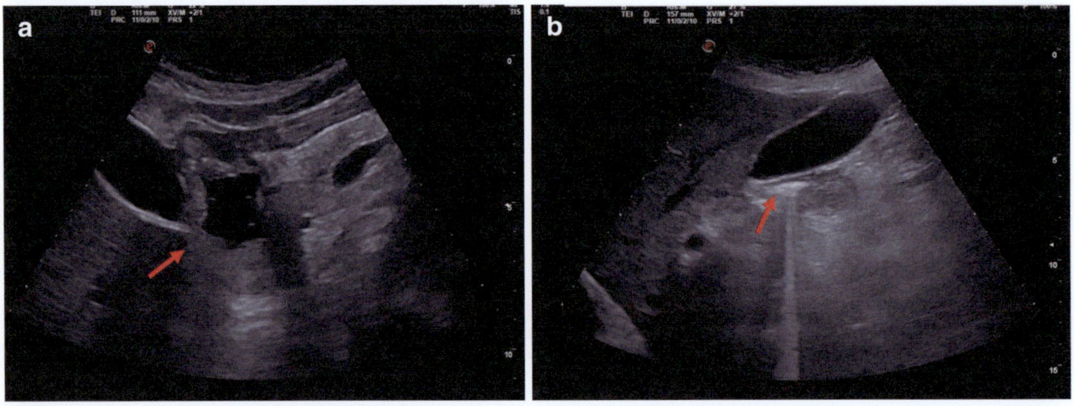

Fig. 1.13 Second portion of the duodenum showing intraluminal fluid in (**a**) and intraluminal gas in (**b**) (arrows)

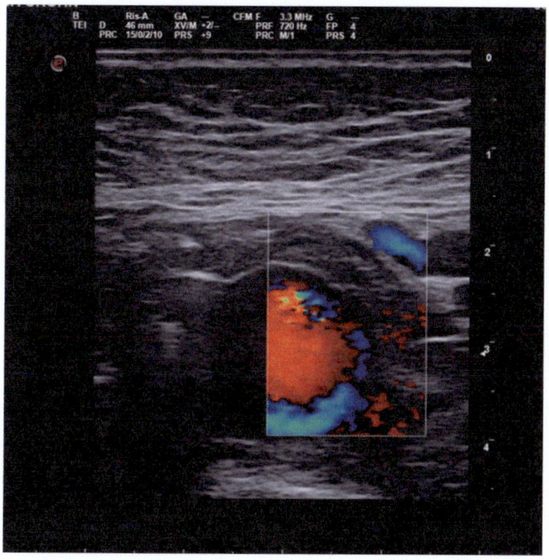

Fig. 1.14 Third portion of the duodenum without endoluminal content, located between the superior mesenteric artery and the aorta

small bowel is performed in two phases. Usually, it includes an overview scanning with the convex probe across the entire abdomen. In the subsequent phase, the detailed assessment using a linear probe is performed with transverse, longitudinal, and oblique scans.

The jejunum is primarily located in the left upper quadrant (LUQ) of the abdomen (Fig. 1.15). Moving toward the terminal ileum in the right iliac fossa, the ileal loops are visible in the meso-hypogastrium and lower right quadrants. In these regions, the folds progressively reduce, ultimately disappearing, and peristaltic activity decreases.

The ileum is visualized using high-frequency linear probes (7.5 MHz) through transverse and oblique scans in the right iliac fossa, applying gradual compression to the abdominal wall to displace any overlapping loops. Anatomical landmarks include the iliopsoas muscle, iliac vessels, and the anterior superior iliac spine. The terminal ileum is located anteromedial to the iliopsoas muscle and medial to the cecum (Fig. 1.16, Video 1.1).

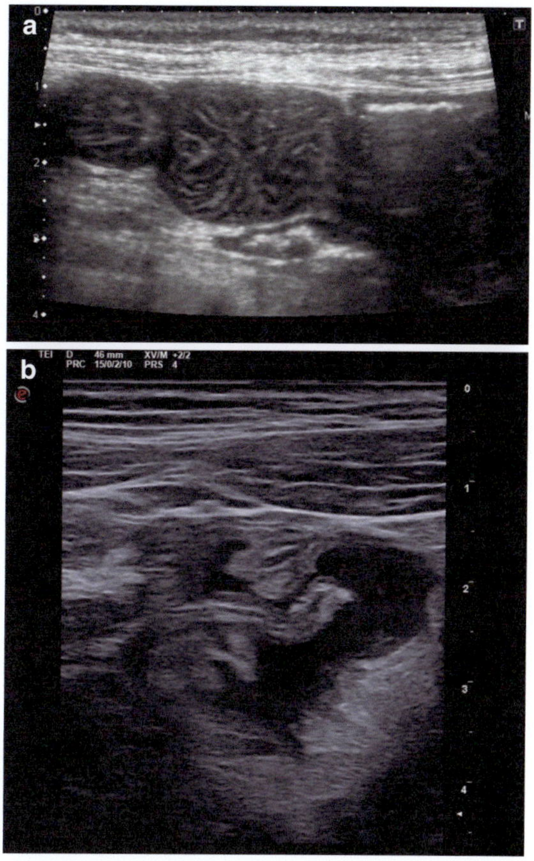

Fig. 1.15 Jejunum without endoluminal content, with multiple folds giving the characteristic cerebriform appearance (**a**). Jejunum with fluid endoluminal content: the Kerckring folds are more clearly visible (**b**)

1.4.5 Appendix

The normal appendix is visualized using high-frequency probes, employing the same landmarks used to identify the terminal ileum and applying similar compression to displace the ileal loops and the cecum in order to reduce artifacts due to their gaseous content. When visible, the normal appendix appears as a thin tubular structure with stratified walls in longitudinal section or rounded in transverse section. It is easily compressible and has a diameter of less than 6 mm. It should be measured including the anterior and posterior walls. It can be distinguished from the terminal ileum by its blind-ending morphology and the absence of peristalsis (Fig. 1.17, Video 1.2).

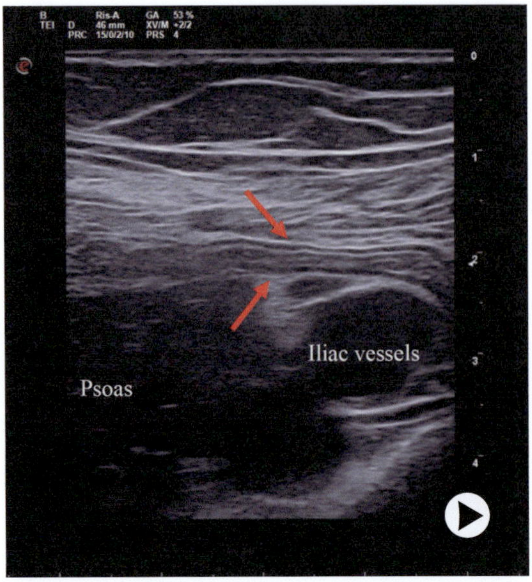

Fig. 1.16 The terminal ileum is visualized anteromedial to the iliac vessels and psoas. Video 1.1 Small bowel (▶ https://doi.org/10.1007/000-j1s)

1.4.6 Colon

The colon is characterized by a higher gas content than the small bowel and a typical haustration, giving it a polycyclic shape.

The ascending colon is detected on the right side, anteromedial to the psoas muscle. The lumen is often distended by air and fecal material, especially in conditions of stasis (Fig. 1.18). The posterior wall, distal to the probe, is often hidden by the intraluminal gas.

The right colic or hepatic flexure is located in the right hypochondrium, below and medial to the liver, anterior to the right kidney (Fig. 1.19).

The transverse colon has a variable position depending on its length and degree of ptosis. It can be located in the epigastrium, mesogastrium, or hypogastrium (ptotic transverse colon). The transverse colon can be observed with longitudinal scans below the gastric antrum. Similarly to

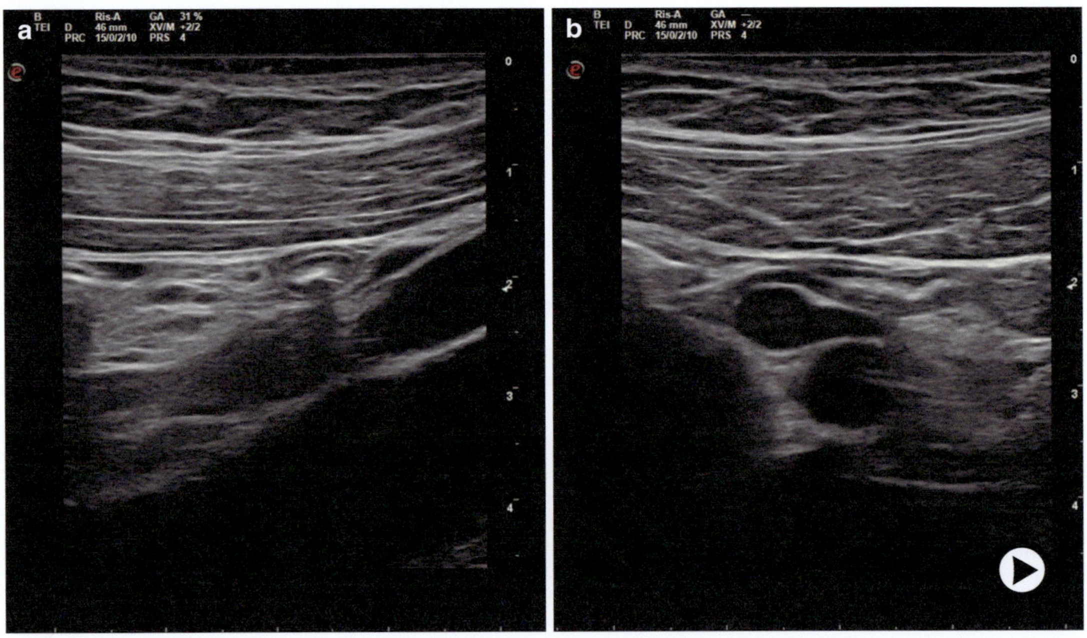

Fig. 1.17 Normal appendix with stratified walls appears as a rounded structure in transverse section (**a**) or as a tubular structure in longitudinal section (**b**)Video 1.2 Appendix (▶ https://doi.org/10.1007/000-j1r)

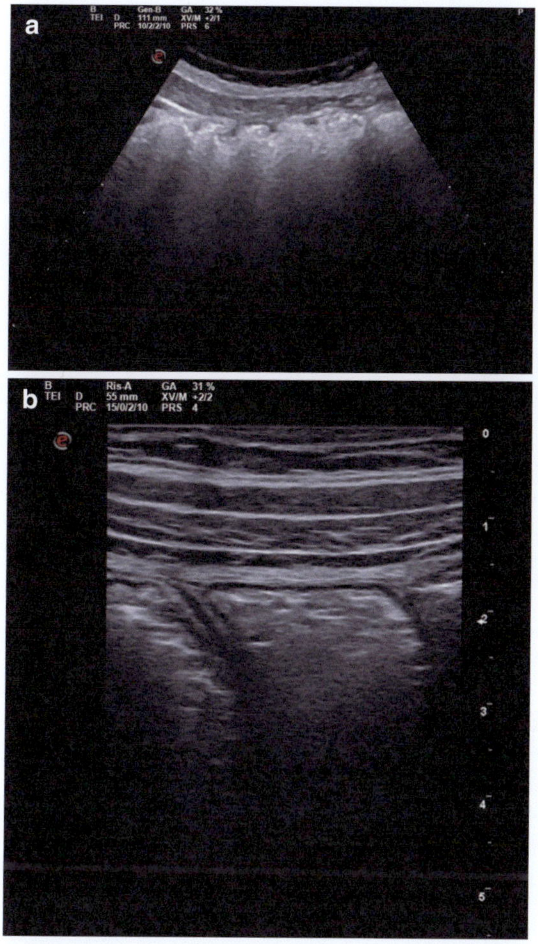

Fig. 1.18 Visualization of the right colon using a convex probe (**a**) and a linear probe (**b**). The characteristic haustrations are more clearly defined using a linear probe

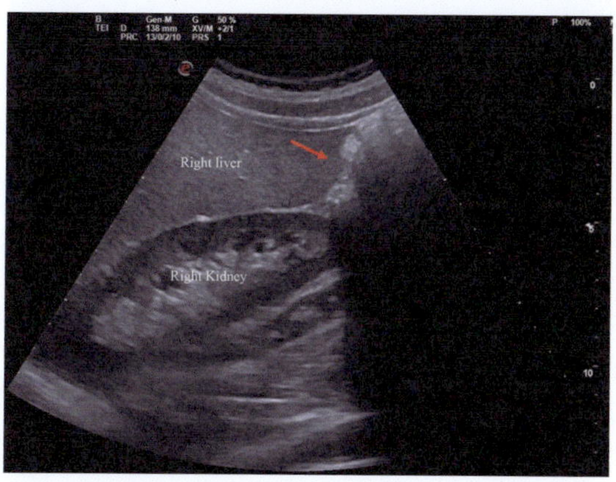

Fig. 1.19 Right colic flexure (arrow) located posterior to the right hepatic lobe, in front of the right kidney

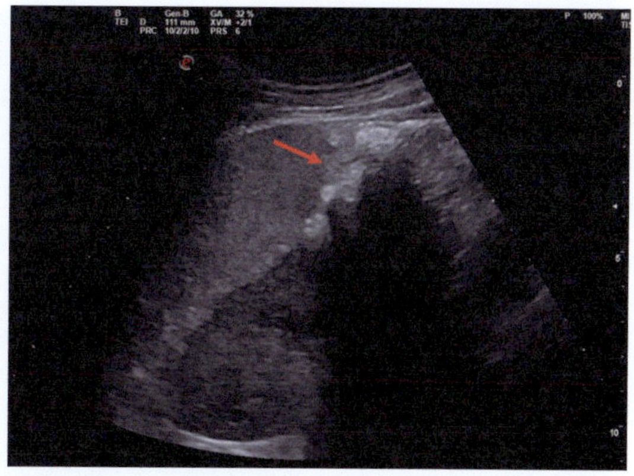

Fig. 1.20 Left colic flexure (arrow) is located adjacent to the inferior pole of the spleen and the left kidney

the right colon, the transverse colon has an undulating profile, is frequently distended by feces, and the posterior wall is not visible.

The left colic or splenic flexure is identified in the left hypochondrium, using a convex probe, with a left intercostal scan (Fig. 1.20).

The descending colon is located on the left side, anteromedial to the psoas muscle. It is less haustrated than the right colon, often appearing contracted and sometimes without luminal content.

The sigmoid colon is located in the left iliac fossa, anterior to the psoas muscle and iliac vessels. Sometimes, the sigmoid colon is located in the right iliac fossa but differs from the terminal ileum due to the absence of peristalsis, the hypertrophy of the muscle layer, and a higher gaseous content (Fig. 1.21).

The sigmoid colon frequently appears contracted and lacks luminal content, allowing visualization of the posterior wall. Due to the hypertrophy of the muscular layer, the sigmdid wall thickness may be normal up to 5 mm (Fig. 1.21).

The rectum is located posterior to the prostate in males and the uterine cervix and vaginal canal in females. In longitudinal scans, it presents a tubular appearance, while in transverse scans, it appears circular. A mild bladder distension can facilitate its visualization (Fig. 1.22).

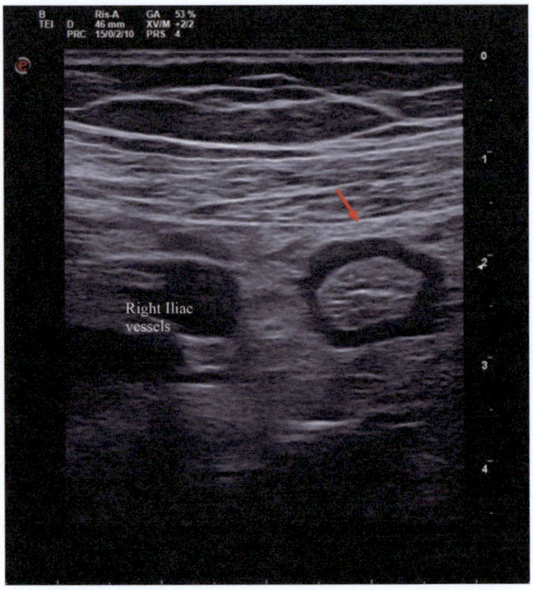

Fig. 1.21 In cases of dolichocolon, the sigmoid colon (red arrow) may be visualized in the right iliac fossa, adjacent to the iliac vessels and the terminal ileum. The hypoechoic muscular layer appears predominant

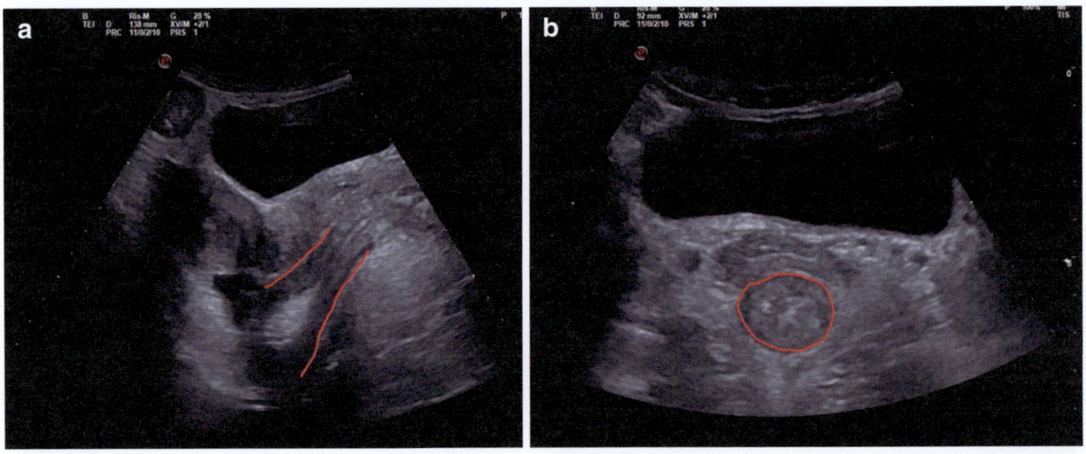

Fig. 1.22 The rectum (red line) appears as a tubular structure in longitudinal scan (**a**) and as a circular structure in transverse scan (**b**)

References

1. Hauser JB, Stanley RJ, Geisse G. The ultrasound findings in an obstructed afferent loop. J Clin Ultrasound. 1974;2:287–9.
2. Daggett PR. Ultrasound in the assessment of intestinal motility. Br J Clin Pract. 1974;28:207–8.
3. Atkinson NSS, Bryant RV, Dong Y, Maaser C, Kucharzik T, Maconi G, Asthana AK, Blaivas M, Goudie A, Gilja OH, Nuernberg D, Schreiber-Dietrich D, Dietrich CF. How to perform gastrointestinal ultrasound: anatomy and normal findings. World J Gastroenterol. 2017;23(38):6931–41.
4. Rapaccini GL, Aliotta A, Pompili M, et al. Gastric wall thickness in normal and neoplastic subjects: a prospective study performed by abdominal ultrasound. Gastrointest Radiol. 1988;13:197–9.
5. Fraquelli M, Colli A, Casazza G, et al. Role of US in detection of Crohn disease: meta-analysis. Radiology. 2005;236:95–101.
6. Su HY, Taylor KM, Friedman AB, Cataletti G, Maconi G. Ultrasound assessment of gastrointestinal luminal contents: a narrative review. J Ultrasound. 2024;27(4):781–92.

Ultrasound in Crohn's Disease: Role of Intestinal Ultrasound in Identifying Crohn's Disease

2

Marta Vernero, Caterina Zoratti, and Cristina Bezzio

Intestinal ultrasound (IUS) is also useful for confirming or excluding the diagnosis of Crohn's disease. As there is no gold standard for the diagnosis of inflammatory bowel disease (IBD), anamnesis, clinical picture, laboratory tests (including faecal calprotectin and C-reactive protein), endoscopy with histological examination, and radiological techniques (IUS and intestinal MRI) are complementary for the diagnosis [1]. Among radiological techniques, IUS is the most manageable as it is usually cheap, easily available, and does not require radiation. In addition, IUS has its highest performance in the terminal ileum, which is the classical location of Crohn's disease. Overall, the sensitivity of IUS in detecting CD is 65.4% and its specificity is 80.5% [2], and its performance is improved by the addition of inflammatory indices such as C-reactive protein and faecal calprotectin [3].

In patients with chronic diarrhoea (especially when unexplained by first-line investigations, including stool culture and Clostridium difficile toxin search), intestinal ultrasound should be performed together with faecal calprotectin to screen patients who need further investigations. Indeed, negative faecal calprotectin together with a normal intestinal ultrasound generally rules out the IBD hypothesis [4]. Bowel wall thickening, loss of bowel wall stratification and echo-pattern, increased bowel wall vascularisation, mesenteric fat thickening, reduction of peristalsis, enlarged lymph nodes, and the presence of free fluid between intestinal loops are the most frequently observed alterations [5]. In addition, complications of Crohn's disease (stenosis, fistulae, abscesses, or inflammatory masses) can be easily detected by means of IUS but will not be discussed in this chapter.

Among the above-mentioned findings in CD, the most important is increased bowel wall thickness (BWT). The final BWT should be reported as the mean of four different measurements of the same bowel segment. Specifically, two measure-

Supplementary Information The online version contains supplementary material available at https://doi.org/10.1007/978-3-032-11418-1_2. The videos can be accessed individually by clicking the DOI link in the accompanying figure caption or by scanning this link with the SN More Media App.

M. Vernero
Division of Gastroenterology, Department of Medical Sciences, University of Turin, Turin, Italy

C. Zoratti
Department of Medical, Surgical and Health Sciences, University of Trieste, Trieste, Italy

C. Bezzio (✉)
IBD Unit, Gastroenterology Department, IRCCS Humanitas Research Hospital, Rozzano, Italy

Department of Biomedical Sciences, Humanitas University, Pieve Emanuele, Italy

F. Terracciano et al. (eds.), *Bowel Ultrasound Compared with Endoscopy*,
https://doi.org/10.1007/978-3-032-11418-1_2

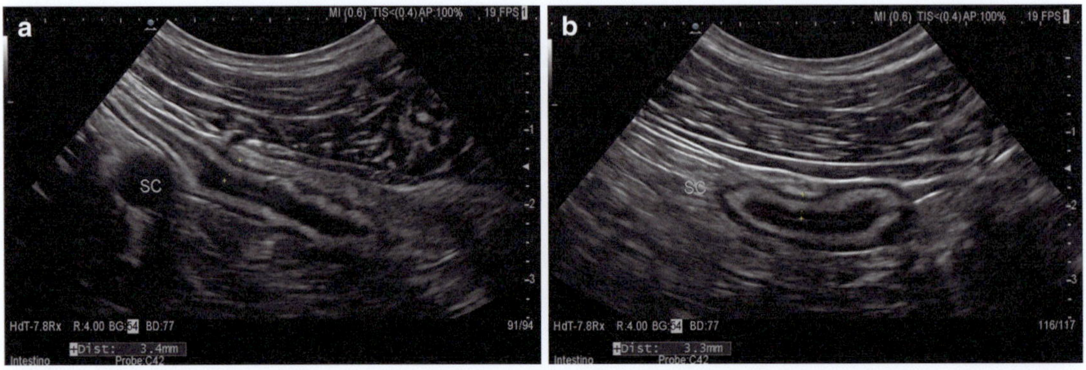

Fig. 2.1 (**a**) Longitudinal scan of the bowel wall thickness of the sigma. (**b**) Transversal scan of the bowel wall thickness of the sigma

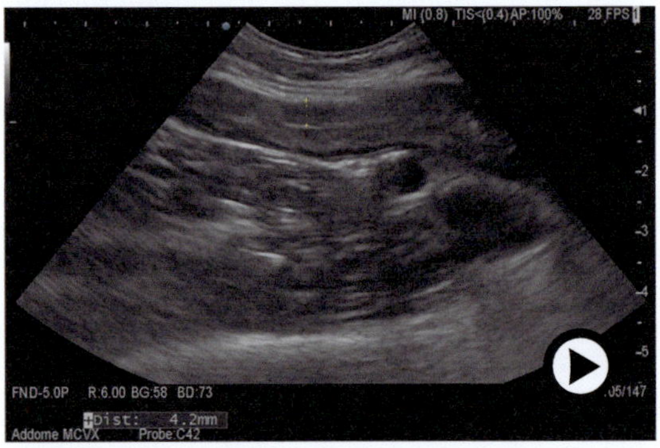

Fig. 2.2 Increased bowel wall thickness with partial loss of stratification over an extension of 15 cm in a patient with ileal Crohn's disease (▶ https://doi.org/10.1007/000-j1v)

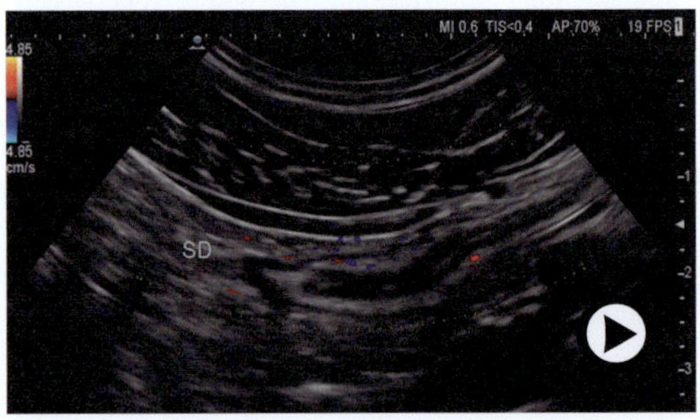

Fig. 2.3 Increased bowel wall thickness, normal stratification, and mild increase of vascularisation (LS 2) of the sigma in patient with Crohn's disease (▶ https://doi.org/10.1007/000-j1t)

ments should be performed in the longitudinal section (at least 1 cm apart) (Fig. 2.1a) and two in the transverse section (at least 90° apart) (Fig. 2.1b). Correct measurement of the BWT should start at the interface between the lumen and mucosa and end at the interface between the muscle and serosa layer, paying attention to keep the calipers perpendicular to the bowel wall [6].

The generally accepted cutoff value for normal bowel wall thickness is 3 mm, both for colon and ileum, taking into account that the duodenal bulb and rectum are normally thicker [7, 8]. However, the cutoff for CD detection is variable, depending on the studies and on the desired balance between sensitivity and specificity. For instance, 3 mm has an 89% sensitivity and a 96% specificity, while 4 mm (or more) has an 87% sensitivity and a 98% specificity. It must be pointed out that these high sensitivity and specificity rates are true for the terminal ileum, while for colonic and ileo-colonic disease only 81% [9] and 91% [10] sensitivity was reached, respectively.

After the detection of a thickened bowel tract, its extension should be estimated (Fig. 2.2). There are still not many studies investigating the accuracy of IUS in measuring the length of the diseased bowel, but some authors found good concordance with X-ray (r = 0.52) and surgical examination (r = 0.64) [11]. When describing a bowel loop, besides its thickness, the stratification of the bowel wall is one of the major characteristics (Fig. 2.3). The bowel wall is made up of five distinct sonographic layers: the first one is hyperechoic and represents the interface between the lumen and the mucosa, the second hypoechoic layer is the mucosa, the third hyperechoic layer corresponds to the submucosa, the fourth hypoechoic layer is composed of the muscular layer, and the last hyperechoic layer (the fifth) represents the interface between the muscular layer and serosa [12]. During an active phase of CD, the bowel wall tends to be completely hypoechoic with no clear distinction between these five layers (Fig. 2.4a). On the contrary, during remission or a phase of chronic inflammation, the stratification is preserved but usually the hyperechoic submucosal layer is more prominent (Fig. 2.4b, c) [13].

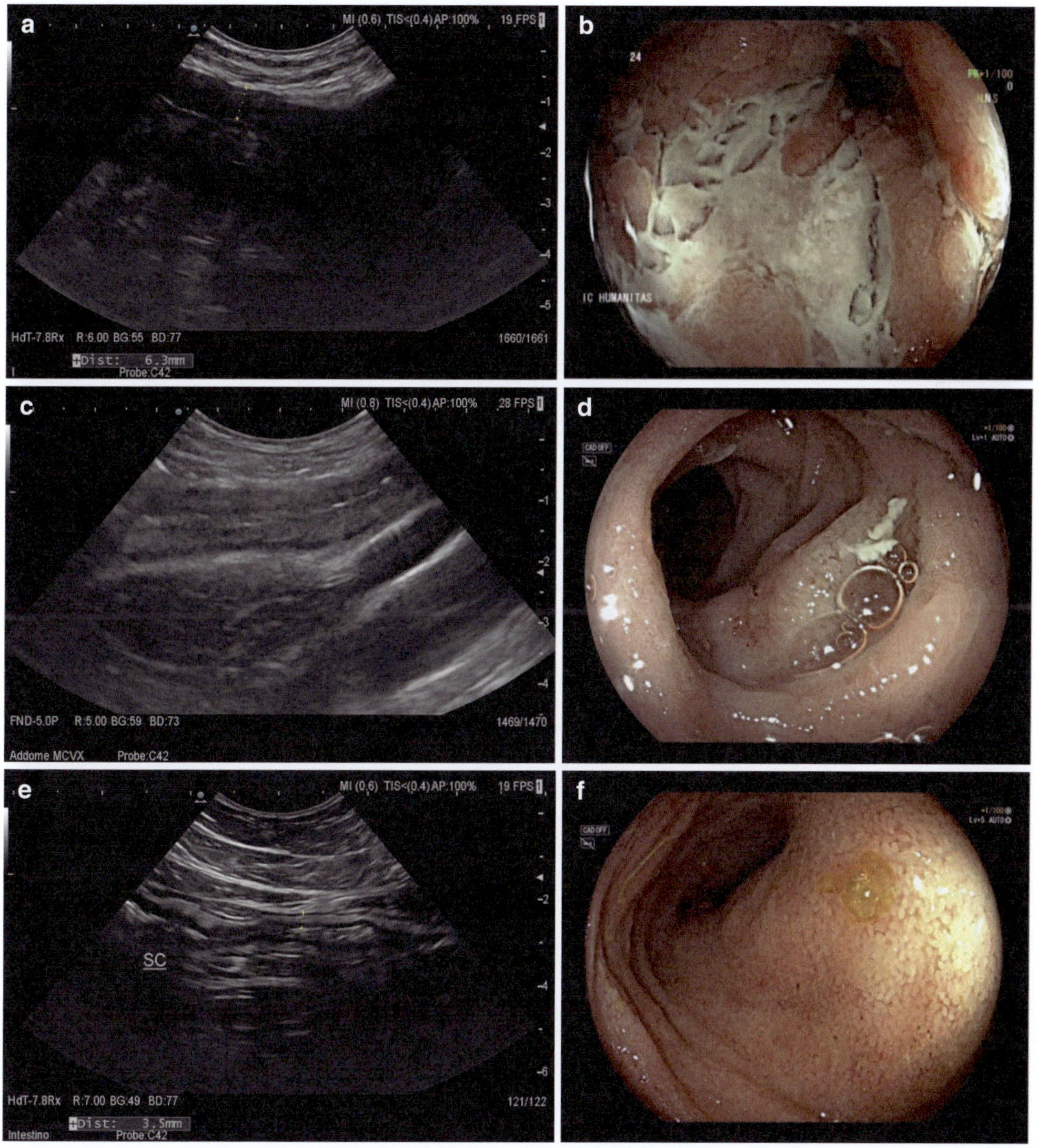

Fig. 2.4 (**a**) Complete loss of bowel wall stratification of the ileum in a patient with Crohn's disease (**b**) Severe ileitis. The endoscopic image corresponds to the ultrasound image shown in Fig. 2.2a. (**c**) Partial loss of bowel wall stratification of the ileum in a patient with Crohn's disease from mild to moderate ileitis (**d**) The endoscopic image corresponds to the ultrasound image shown in Fig. 2.2c. (**e**) Normal stratification of the bowel wall of the sigma in a patient with Crohn's disease. (**f**) Endoscopic remission. The endoscopic image corresponds to a normal ultrasound image with BWT <3 mm and normal stratification of the bowel wall of the ileum

Another fundamental aspect of the bowel wall to be evaluated is the vascularisation, usually evaluated through Colour Doppler evaluation, although this is a very poorly standardised method [14]. For this purpose, an activity score was created, called the Limberg score (Fig. 2.5). According to this score, grade 0 means that there is no bowel wall thickening or vascularisation (normal BWT); grade 1 means bowel wall thickening greater than 3 mm without vascularisation (Fig. 2.6a); grade 2 means bowel wall thickening with some spots of vascularity (Fig. 2.6b); grade 3 stands for bowel wall thickening with long stretches of vascularity (Fig. 2.6c); and grade

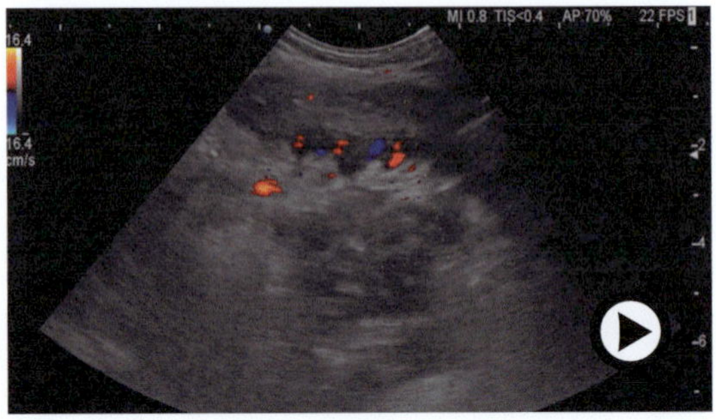

Fig. 2.5 Increased vascularisation (LS 2–3) of the terminal ileum in a patient with Crohn's disease (▶ https://doi.org/10.1007/000-j1w)

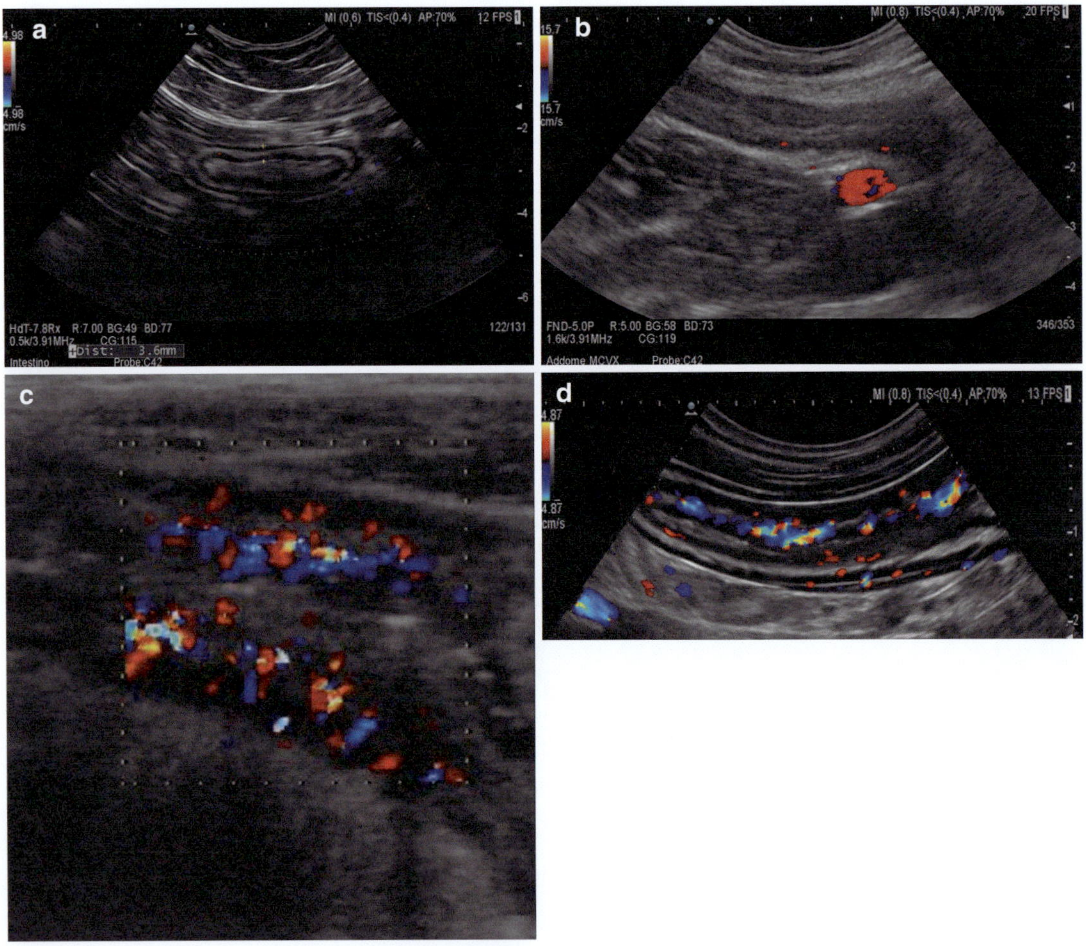

Fig. 2.6 (**a**) Limberg score grade 1: bowel wall thickening greater than 3 mm without vascularisation. (**b**) Limberg score grade 2: bowel wall thickening with some spots of vascularity. (**c**) Limberg score grade 3: bowel wall thickening with long stretches of vascularity. (**d**) Limberg score grade 4: bowel wall thickening with long stretches of vascularity extending into the mesentery

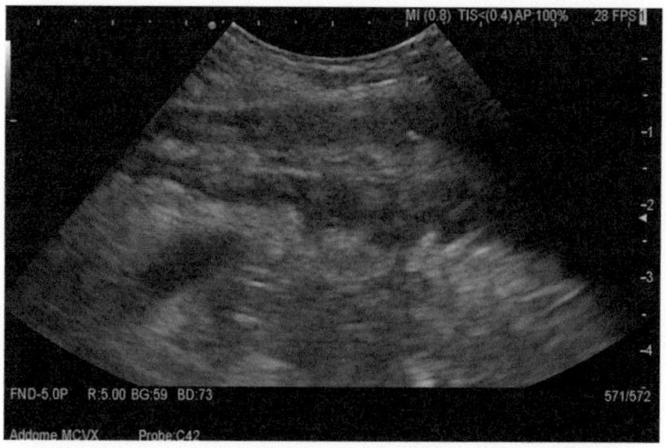

Fig. 2.7 Irregularities of the external and internal margins of the bowel wall of the ileum in a patient with Crohn's disease

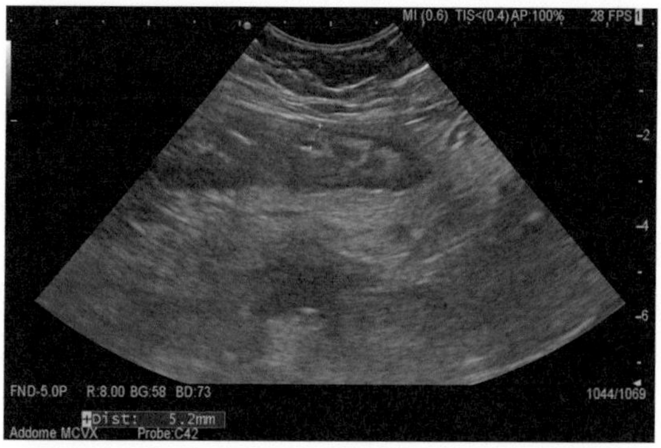

Fig. 2.8 Hypertrophy of mesenteric fat in a patient with Crohn's disease

4 indicates bowel wall thickening with long stretches of vascularity extending into the mesentery (Fig. 2.6d) [15].

Further aspects to be investigated include irregularities of the external and internal margins (Fig. 2.7), often indicating possible deep ulcers or early fistulas; ulcers may also be observed between layers [5]. Moreover, some extra-intestinal aspects may be investigated to support the diagnosis of Crohn's disease, such as the hypertrophy of mesenteric fat (Fig. 2.8), the presence of enlarged mesenteric lymph nodes (Fig. 2.9), or the presence of free fluid between the intestinal loops [5].

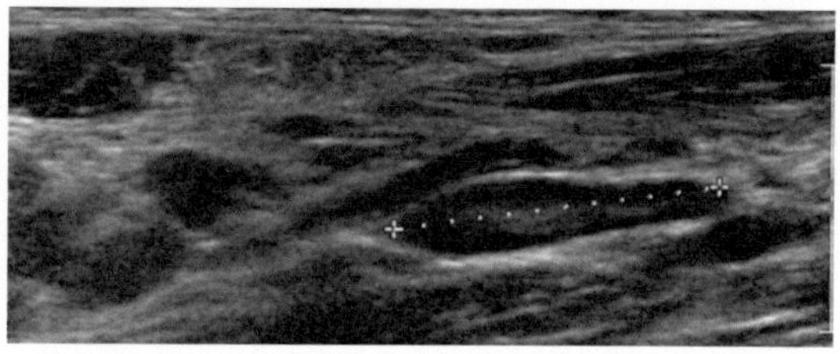

Fig. 2.9 Enlarged mesenteric lymph node in a patient with Crohn's disease

References

1. Maaser C, Sturm A, Vavricka SR, et al. ECCO-ESGAR Guideline for Diagnostic Assessment in IBD Part 1: Initial diagnosis, monitoring of known IBD, detection of complications. J Crohns Colitis. 2019;13:144–64.
2. Panes J, Bouhnik Y, Reinisch W, et al. Imaging techniques for assessment of inflammatory bowel disease: joint ECCO and ESGAR evidence-based consensus guidelines. J Crohns Colitis. 2013;7:556–85.
3. Paredes JM, Ripollés T, Algarra Á, Diaz R, Moreno N, Latorre P, Martínez MJ, Llopis P, López A, Moreno-Osset E. Intestinal ultrasonography and fecal calprotectin for monitoring inflammation of ileal Crohn's disease: two complementary tests. Intest Res. 2022;20:361–9.
4. Fraquelli M, Colli A, Casazza G, Paggi S, Colucci A, Massironi S, Duca P, Conte D. Role of US in detection of Crohn disease: meta-analysis. Radiology. 2005;236:95–101.
5. Fraquelli M, Castiglione F, Calabrese E, Maconi G. Impact of intestinal ultrasound on the management of patients with inflammatory bowel disease: how to apply scientific evidence to clinical practice. Dig Liver Dis Off J Ital Soc Gastroenterol Ital Assoc Study Liver. 2020;52:9–18.
6. Maaser C, Maconi G, Kucharzik T, Allocca M. Ultrasonography in inflammatory bowel disease – so far we are? United Eur Gastroenterol J. 2022;10:225–32.
7. Huh CH, Bhutani MS, Farfán EB, Bolch WE. Individual variations in mucosa and total wall thickness in the stomach and rectum assessed via endoscopic ultrasound. Physiol Meas. 2003;24:N15–22.
8. Nylund K, Hausken T, Ødegaard S, Eide GE, Gilja OH. Gastrointestinal wall thickness measured with transabdominal ultrasonography and its relationship to demographic factors in healthy subjects. Ultraschall Med Stuttg Ger 1980. 2012;33:E225–32.
9. Maconi G, Parente F, Bollani S, Cesana B, Bianchi Porro G. Abdominal ultrasound in the assessment of extent and activity of Crohn's disease: clinical significance and implication of bowel wall thickening. Am J Gastroenterol. 1996;91:1604–9.

10. Hirche TO, Russler J, Schröder O, Schuessler G, Kappeser P, Caspary WF, Dietrich CF. The value of routinely performed ultrasonography in patients with Crohn disease. Scand J Gastroenterol. 2002;37:1178–83.
11. Parente F, Maconi G, Bollani S, Anderloni A, Sampietro G, Cristaldi M, Franceschelli N, Bianco R, Taschieri AM, Bianchi Porro G. Bowel ultrasound in assessment of Crohn's disease and detection of related small bowel strictures: a prospective comparative study versus x ray and intraoperative findings. Gut. 2002;50:490–5.
12. Nylund K, Maconi G, Hollerweger A, et al. EFSUMB recommendations and guidelines for gastrointestinal ultrasound. Ultraschall Med Stuttg Ger 1980. 2017;38:273–84.
13. Allocca M, Craviotto V, Dell'Avalle C, Furfaro F, Zilli A, D'Amico F, Bonovas S, Peyrin-Biroulet L, Fiorino G, Danese S. Bowel ultrasound score is accurate in assessing response to therapy in patients with Crohn's disease. Aliment Pharmacol Ther. 2022;55:446–54.
14. Schwerk WB, Beckh K, Raith M. A prospective evaluation of high resolution sonography in the diagnosis of inflammatory bowel disease. Eur J Gastroenterol Hepatol. 1992:173–82.
15. Limberg B. Diagnosis of chronic inflammatory bowel disease by ultrasonography. Z Gastroenterol. 1999;37:495–508.

Role of IUS in the Assessment of Disease Activity and Response-to-Treatment in Crohn's Disease

3

Fabrizio Santagata, Nicole Piazza O Sed, and Mirella Fraquelli

3.1 Introduction

The use of IUS has become a widely accepted tool for monitoring Crohn's disease. IUS is a quick-to-run and readily available technique, which can provide responses in real-time and support early clinical decision-making in routine IBD (inflammatory bowel disease) care [1].

Among the parameters assessed to evaluate disease activity, the degree of bowel-wall thickness (BWT) is the primary and most relevant finding as it has been shown to correlate with endoscopic activity and clinical symptoms [1–5].

Supplementary Information The online version contains supplementary material available at https://doi.org/10.1007/978-3-032-11418-1_3. The videos can be accessed individually by clicking the DOI link in the accompanying figure caption or by scanning this link with the SN More Media App.

F. Santagata
Department of Pathophysiology and Transplantation, University of Milan, Milan, Italy

N. P. O Sed
Gastroenterology and Endoscopy Unit, Fondazione IRCCS Ca' Granda Ospedale Maggiore Policlinico, Milan, Italy

M. Fraquelli (✉)
Gastroenterology and Endoscopy Unit, Fondazione IRCCS Ca' Granda Ospedale Maggiore Policlinico, Milan, Italy
e-mail: mirella.fraquelli@policlinico.mi.it

In adult IBD patients, a BWT cutoff value >3 mm is the most consistent single IUS parameter correlating with endoscopic activity [6, 7].

In addition, active Crohn's disease is associated with the appearance of neoangiogenesis as documented by anatomopathological studies, angiographic findings, and by the presence of angiogenic factors in the serum of patients with active Crohn's [8]. Therefore, after BWT, the evidence of hyperemia at color Doppler imaging (CDI) represents another critical parameter for assessing disease activity. This is achieved through specialized presets optimized for detecting slow blood flow. Indeed, color Doppler flow is usually semi-quantitative and subjectively graded. The subjective assessment of vascularity by IUS suggests that vessel density reflects inflammatory activity [6, 9].

Bowel-wall vascularity seems to be correlated with endoscopic activity [2], clinical activity [10] and to a lesser extent, with biochemical markers such as C-reactive protein (CRP) and fecal calprotectin (FC) [11].

When combined with increased BWT, increased hyperemia is almost always representative of active disease. Indeed, most studies aimed at developing IUS scores to predict disease activity, using endoscopy as the reference standard, have demonstrated through multivariate analyses that the only independent predictors of endoscopic activity are BWT and hyperemia [12–15].

F. Terracciano et al. (eds.), *Bowel Ultrasound Compared with Endoscopy*,
https://doi.org/10.1007/978-3-032-11418-1_3

The bowel-wall echopattern has also been proposed as a valuable parameter for identifying active disease. Specifically, focal disruption of bowel wall layers and a hypoechoic pattern with loss of bowel-wall stratification have been reported to be more prevalent in patients with active disease, whereas a stratified pattern is more commonly observed in those with inactive disease [16].

Among the additional features of inflammation in IBD are inflammatory mesenteric fat wrapping (creeping fat), which appears as hyperechoic encasing of the inflamed bowel, the presence of free fluid within the bowel loops, and enlarged mesenteric lymph nodes [17].

To date, numerous ultrasonographic activity scores have been proposed for assessing disease activity in Crohn's disease using several and often combined IUS parameters. However, only a few of these scoring systems have undergone formal validation.

Contrast-enhanced ultrasound (CEUS) involves the intravenous injection of stabilized microbubbles of small gas particles containing sulfur hexafluoride (2–6 μm) to increase the backscatter signal from blood cells [17–19].

Following the identification of a region of interest (ROI) within the thickened bowel segment, the subsequent enhancement is recorded as a continuous cine-loop file for 100 seconds immediately after contrast injection, without requiring breath-holding. The software then automatically generates multiple parameters related to blood flow and volume by analyzing the time-intensity curve. From this analysis, the following parameters can be derived and assessed: maximum gradient, maximum gradient time, mean gradient to the peak, arrival time, time to peak intensity, peak intensity, time width at half maximum, time width ratio, area under the curve, wash-in area under the curve, and wash-out area under the curve [20, 21].

Several primary studies and meta-analyses have demonstrated that the presence of bowel-wall enhancement on CEUS is associated with significant inflammation, whereas its absence shows high accuracy in excluding active disease [20–25]. However, the evidence supporting the routine use of CEUS remains limited, as the available studies are based on small cohorts and exhibit considerable methodological heterogeneity. To implement effectively the method in everyday practice, it is necessary to conduct a comprehensive prospective study on the role of CEUS in active CD detection.

3.2 Assessment of Crohn's Disease Activity

3.2.1 Clinical Scenario 1: Assessment of Ileal Disease

A 73-year-old woman with clinically silent extensive ileal Crohn's disease (A3-L1-B2 according to Montreal) was admitted to the GI department for deterioration of her general condition and weight loss. The IUS test performed at admission showed extensive bowel-wall thickening (Figs. 3.1 and 3.2; Video 3.1) of the terminal ileum; loss of layer stratification with tendency to hypoechogenicity (Fig. 3.3), grade-3 hypervascularity according to the Limberg score (Fig. 3.4, Table 3.1), and an IBUS-SAS score of 72, suggesting moderate to severe endoscopic activity (Table 3.2). Upon evaluation with a convex probe, the presence of free fluid between the bowel loops, mesenteric hypertrophy, and reactive lymphadenopathy were also observed (Figs. 3.5 and 3.6). Endoscopic evaluation to assess the extent and severity of the ileal disease was not feasible due to the presence of a stenotic ileocecal valve that could not be traversed with a standard colonoscope (Figs. 3.7 and 3.8).

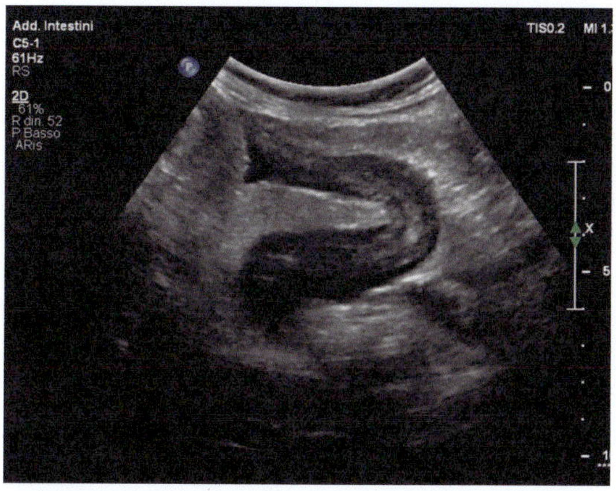

Fig. 3.1 IUS. Extended proximal ileal tract with BWT and prevalently hypoechoic pattern surrounded by hypertrophic and activated mesentery

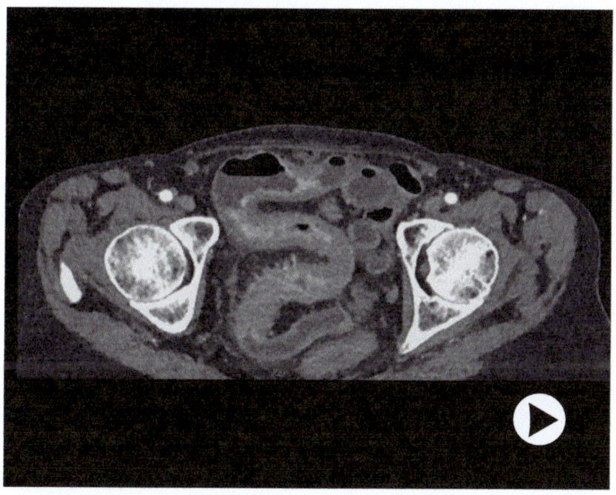

Fig. 3.2 CT enterography showing extensive thickening of the terminal ileum. The fat halo sign can be observed, demonstrating three bowel wall layers: soft-tissue density of inner and outer layers, with interspersed layer of fatty density, sign of chronic inflammationVideo 3.1 Entero-CT vs IUS for evaluating ileal Crohn's disease (▶ https://doi.org/10.1007/000-j1y)

3.2.2 Clinical Scenario 2: Assessment of Colonic Disease Activity

The patient is a 63-year-old woman affected by colonic Crohn's disease (A3-L2-B1 according to Montreal), on infliximab therapy for steroid refractory disease. Despite mild control of symptoms, the follow-up colonoscopy repeated after 1

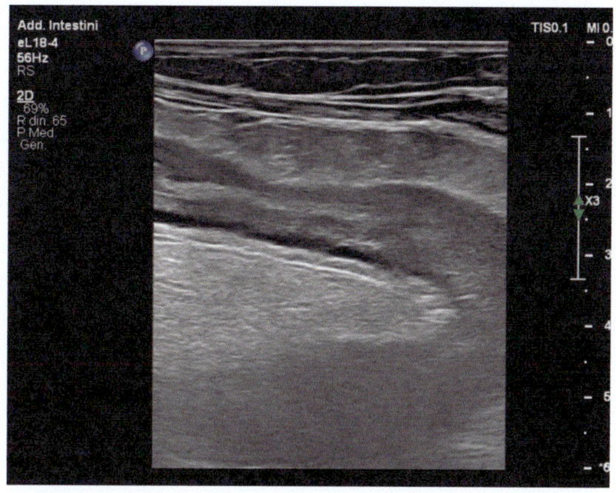

Fig. 3.3 IUS. Crohn's disease. Mid-proximal ileal tract with thickened bowel wall with a prevalently hypoechoic pattern and partially lost bowel wall stratification. Mesenteric hypertrophy surrounding the bowel tract

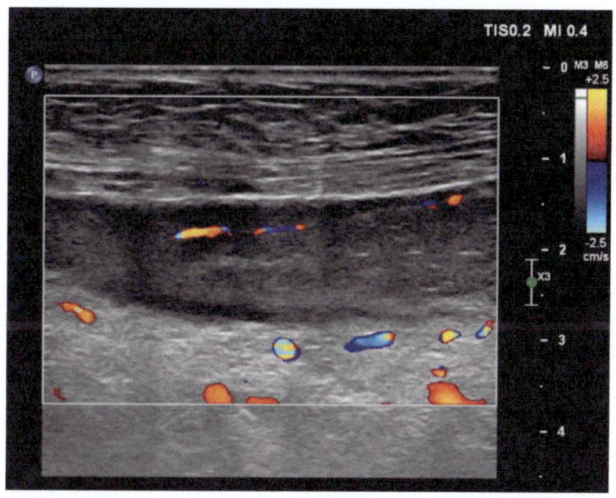

Fig. 3.4 IUS. Particular of Fig. 3.3 showing a mid-proximal ileal tract with increased vascularization at CDI in the bowel wall and in the surrounding mesentery

year on infliximab therapy showed persistent involvement of the transverse and left colon, characterized by wide, deep ulcers. A SES-CD score above 20 was recorded (Figs. 3.9, 3.10, and 3.11; Video 3.2). The IUS showed good agreement with endoscopy, showing bowel-wall thickening, with marked over-representation of the hyperechoic submucosal layer from the hepatic flexure to the sigmoid colon (Figs. 3.10, 3.12, 3.13, and 3.14). CDI signals demonstrated grade-3 hypervascularization according to the Limberg score (Figs. 3.14, 3.15, and 3.16).

Table 3.1 The Limberg Scoring System for US assessment of Crohn's disease activity [26][a]

Grade	Features
1	No vascularization signal at color Doppler imaging
2	Mild: minimal signal, short stretches on vascularization spots
3	Moderate: longer stretches of vascularity, blood vessels are only intra-murally located
4	Severe: long continuous intra- and extra-mural blood vessels, extending into the mesentery

[a]Limberg scoring system (Grades 1–4) for intestinal ultrasound assessment of Crohn's disease activity using color Doppler.Grades reflect increasing mural vascularity, from absent signal (Grade 1) to marked continuous intra- and extramural flow. Severe grades include extension of vascular signals beyond the bowel wall into the mesentery. The score is applied to the most affected segment to support standardized grading and follow-up [26]

Table 3.2 The IBUS-SAS Scoring System for US assessment of Crohn's disease activity [27][a]

	0	1	2	3
BWT	≤3 mm	/	>3 mm	/
i-fat	Absent	Uncertain	Present	/
CDS	Absent	Short signals	Long signal inside bowel	Long signal inside and outside the bowel
BWS	Normal	Uncertain	Focal (≤3 cm)	Extensive (>3 cm)

IBUS-SAS (0–100) = 4 × BWT + 15 × i-fat + 7 × CDS + 4 × BWS

BWT bowel wall thickness, *i-fat* inflammatory fat, *CDS* color Doppler signal, *BWS* bowel wall stratification

[a]IBUS-SAS (International Bowel Ultrasound Segmental Activity Score) criteria for ultrasound assessment of Crohn's disease activity. The score integrates bowel wall thickness (BWT), inflammatory fat (i-fat), color Doppler signal (CDS), and extent of bowel wall involvement (BWS) into ordinal categories (0–3). Defined cut-offs and qualitative descriptors aim to standardize segmental reporting and improve comparability across examinations [27]

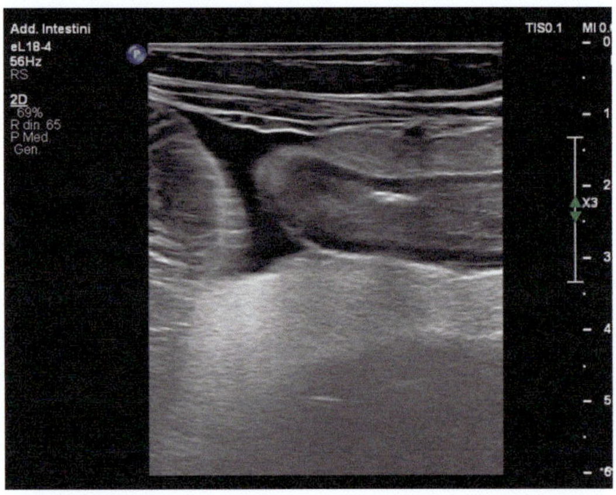

Fig. 3.5 IUS. Free fluid within the bowel loops and mesenteric activation

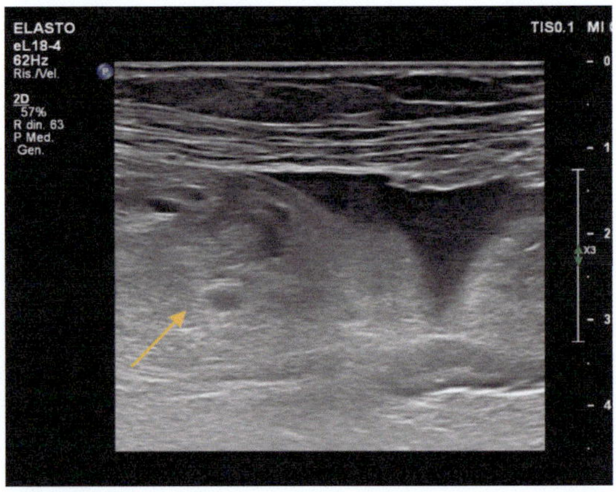

Fig. 3.6 IUS. Multiple enlarged lymph nodes

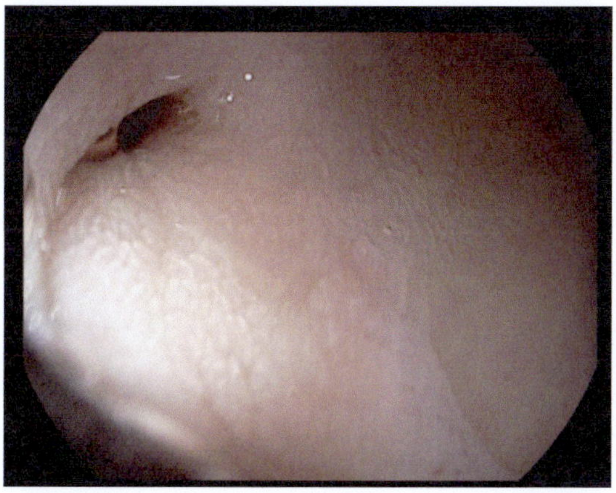

Fig. 3.7 Endoscopy. Ileocecal valve stenosis that could not be passed using a colonoscope

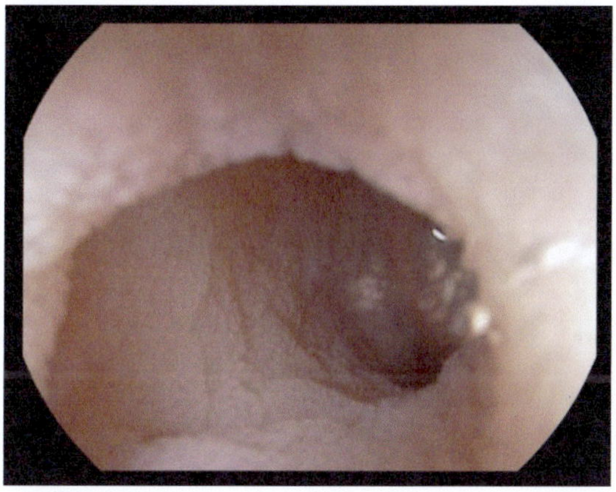

Fig. 3.8 Endoscopic view of the terminal ileum through the stenotic ileocecal valve, no apparent signs of mucosal activity (ulcers, aphthae, erosions)

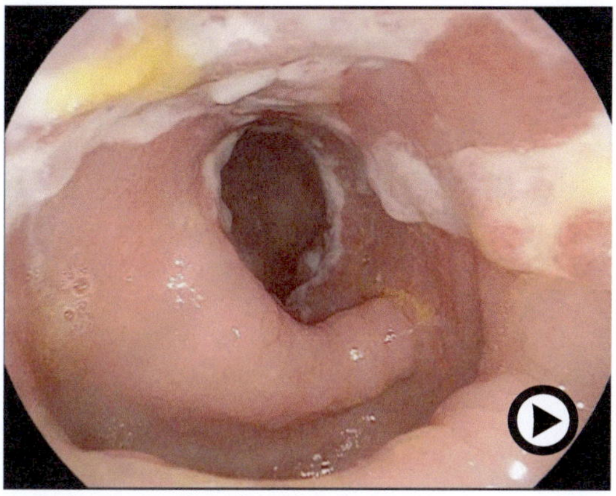

Fig. 3.9 Endoscopy. Transverse colon ulcers, severe endoscopic activityVideo 3.2 Correlation between endoscopic and transmural activity in colonic Crohn's disease (▶ https://doi.org/10.1007/000-j1x)

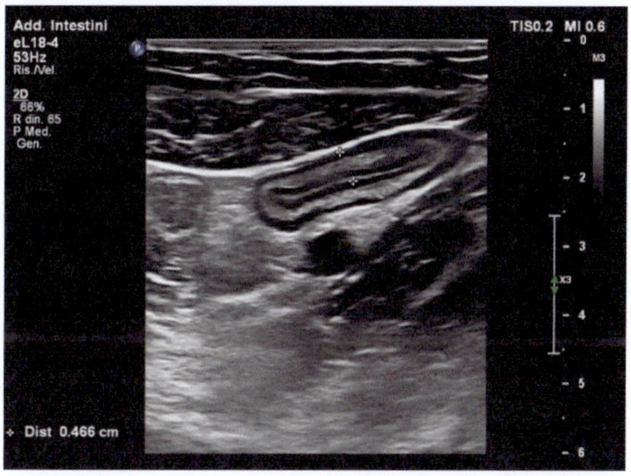

Fig. 3.10 Sigmoid colon with BWT (4.6 mm) with maintained layer stratification and without luminal content

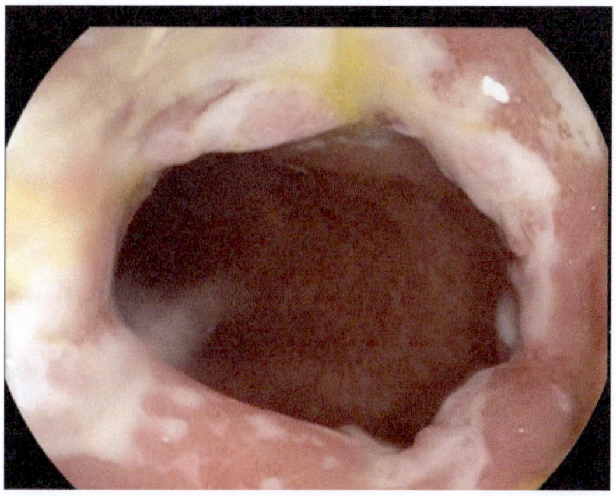

Fig. 3.11 Endoscopy. Ulcerated stricture of the descending colon, upstream revealing a patchy mucosal sparing, a distinctive feature of colonic Crohn's disease

3.2.3 Clinical Scenario 3: Comparison with Other Imaging Techniques: Magnetic Resonance Enterography (MRE)

The patient is 42-year-old diagnosed with ileocecal Crohn's disease treated with infliximab since diagnosis. A recent colonoscopy reveals a traversable ileocecal stenosis with signs of moderate activity, evidenced by ulcers and hyperemia (Fig. 3.17).

Diagnostic imaging, including IUS (Figs. 3.18 and 3.19) and enteric MRI (Fig. 3.20), shows the thickening of the bowel wall of the terminal

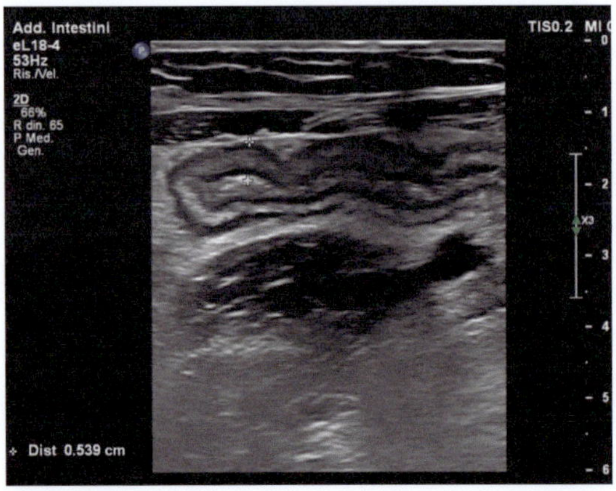

Fig. 3.12 IUS. Transverse colon with BWT (5.2 mm) with maintained layer stratification and hypertrophic submucosa

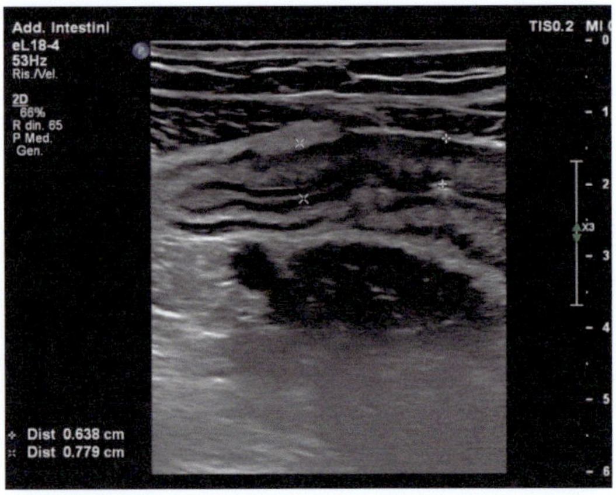

Fig. 3.13 IUS. Sigmoid colon with BWT (up to 7 mm) with maintained stratification and increased submucosal layer

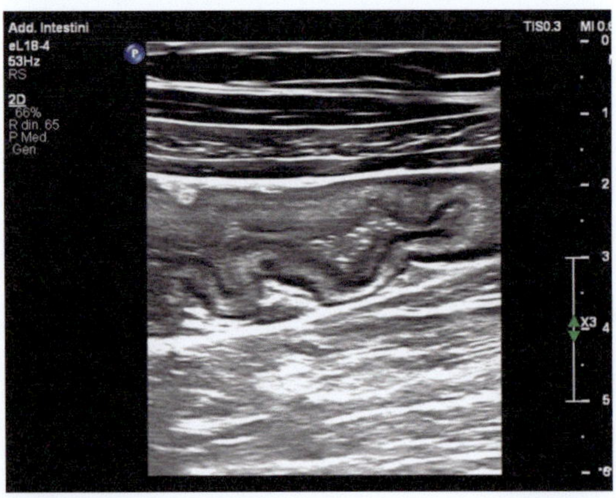

Fig. 3.14 IUS. Descending colon with BWT and maintained stratification

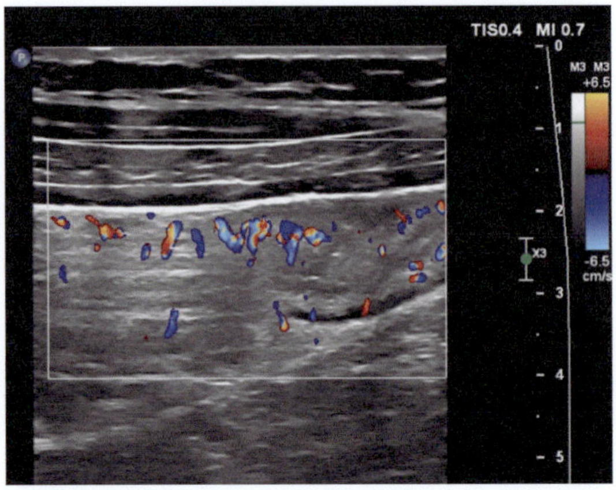

Fig. 3.15 IUS. Sigmoid colon with increased bowel wall vascularization at CDI (Limberg score 3)

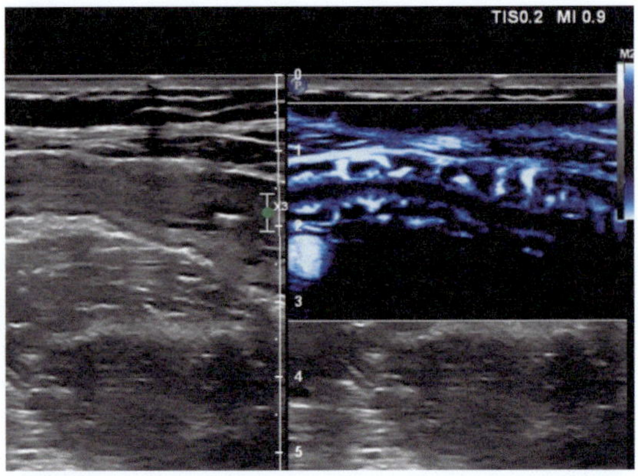

Fig. 3.16 IUS. Descending colon with increased bowel-wall vascularization at microflow imaging with color power angio (CPA) imaging

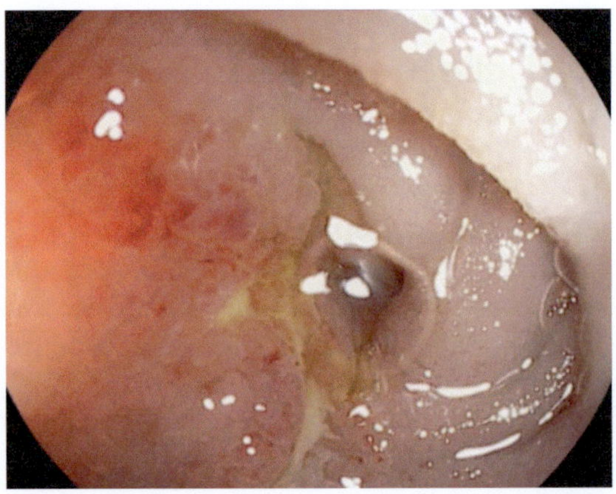

Fig. 3.17 Endoscopic view of the ileal stenosis non-passable by a normal colonoscope. Hyperemia and ulcers can be observed at the distal margin of the stenosis

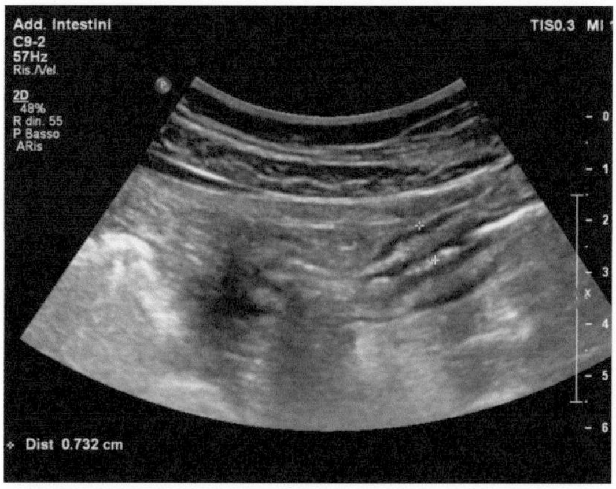

Fig. 3.18 IUS. Thickening of the terminal ileum with altered wall stratification, resulting in submucosal layer hypertrophy

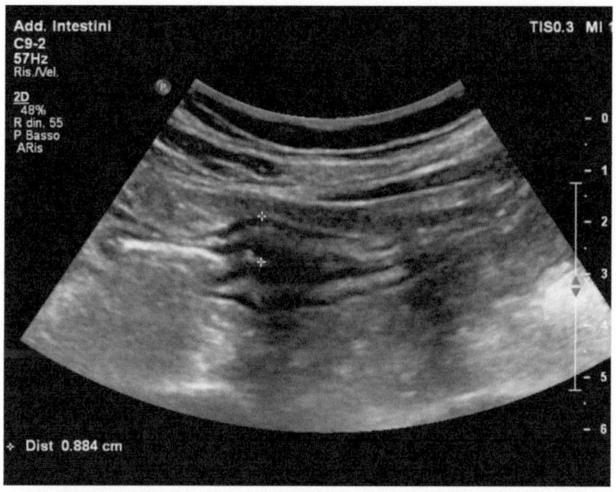

Fig. 3.19 Pathological thickening of the terminal ileum up to 8 mm, along with the concomitant presence of hypoechoic mesenteric tissue surrounding the bowel loop

ileum tract up to 8 mm (Figs. 3.18, 3.19, 3.20, and 3.21), with an approximate extension of 6 cm (Fig. 3.21) and mild upstream dilation (Fig. 3.22).

3.2.4 Clinical Scenario 4: Microvascular CPA (Color Power Angio) in Mild Disease

The patient is a 57-year-old man affected by ileocecal Crohn's disease since 2004 (A2-L3-B2 according to Montreal). After the development of a steroid-dependent disease, combo therapy with azathioprine and infliximab was started in 2015.

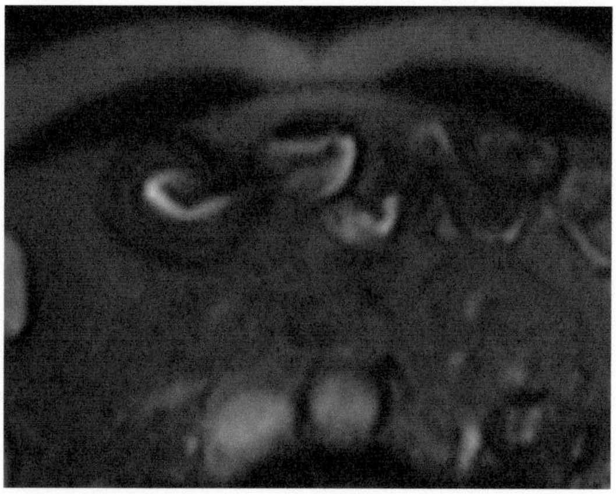

Fig. 3.20 MRI enterography showing BWT of an ileal segment with contrast enhancement of the mucosal layer of the stenosis during the arterial phase. Relative contrast enhancement is one of the items used to assess disease activity in radiological scores such as, e.g., the Magnetic Resonance Index of Activity (MaRIA)

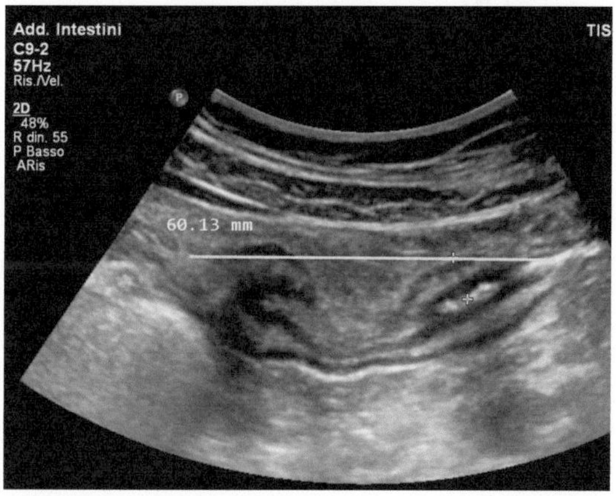

Fig. 3.21 Measuring the extension of bowel-wall thickening using a low-frequency convex probe can be beneficial as reducing the error rates compared to using a linear probe

The ultrasound images show a mild ileal wall thickening with a preserved layer stratification (Figs. 3.23, 3.24, and 3.25). Despite the absence of detectable signals at color Doppler analysis, mild signs of active disease were shown on color power angio (CPA) imaging (Fig. 3.24). Assessing the microvascular flow can be useful to detect mild signs of active disease and helpful in discriminating between inflammation and fibrosis. The ultrasonographic findings are consistent

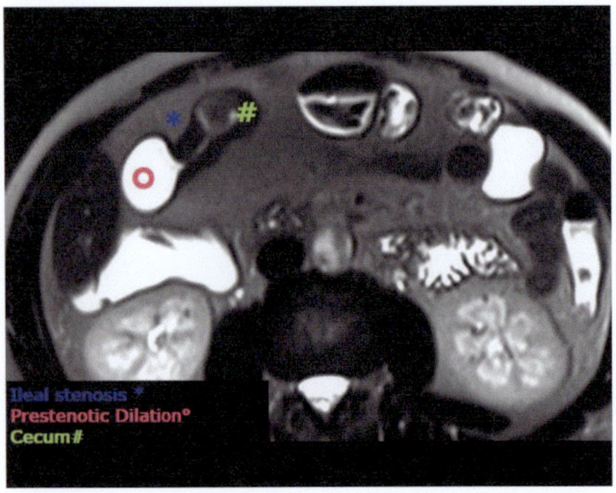

Fig. 3.22 T2 MRI enterography, terminal ileum stenosis (*) resulting in pre-stenotic dilatation of bowel loop

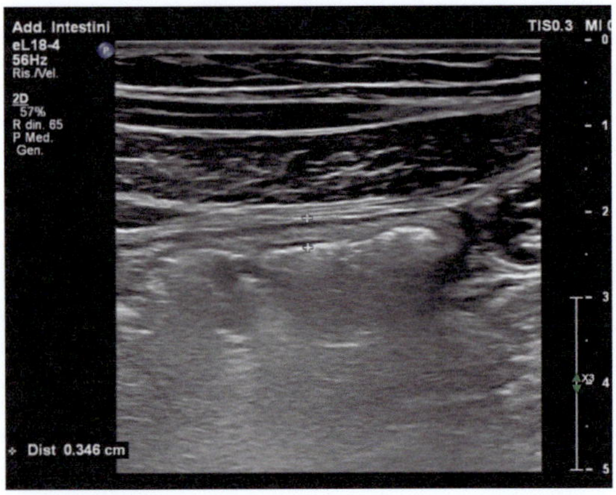

Fig. 3.23 IUS. Mild thickening of the ileal wall with preserved layer stratification is clearly visible in this image. The integrity of the distinct layers is maintained, despite the overall increase in wall thickness

with the endoscopic ones, indicating mild disease at the level of the ileum (Fig. 3.26).

3.2.5 Clinical Scenario 5: Shear Wave Elastography in Defining Disease Activity

The patient is a 17-year-old man with a recent diagnosis of ileocecal Crohn's disease (A1-L3-B3p). The main issue at presentation was represented by perianal disease, apparently in the absence of rectal involvement at endoscopic assessment. The young man complained of bloody diarrhea (eight bowel movements a day) and persistent perianal drainage. At the first ultrasound evaluation bowel-wall thickening of the cecum and appendix were found, with ulcers and loss of layer stratification with marked hypoechogenicity (Figs. 3.27 and 3.28) and hypervascularity in both the bowel wall and the adjacent mesenteric fat (Figs. 3.29 and 3.30). Shear wave elastography (2D-SWE) showed increased bowel-wall stiffness (Fig. 3.31).

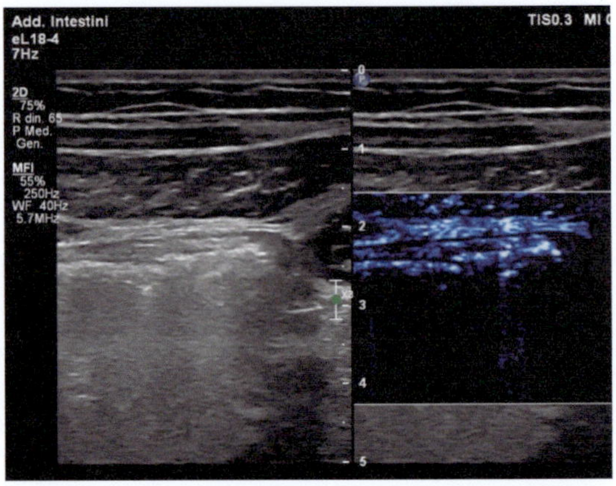

Fig. 3.24 IUS. Despite no detection of signals on color Doppler analysis, mild signs of active disease were shown with micro CPA analysis (color power angio), which is a Doppler technique that allows visualization of low-velocity microcirculation

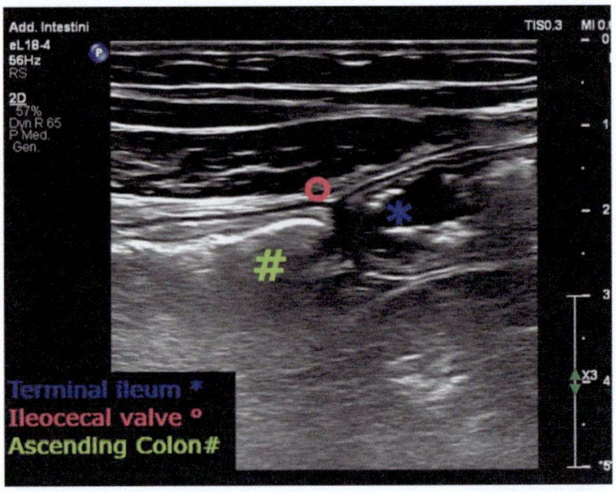

Fig. 3.25 IUS. Longitudinal scan showing mild ileal thickening at the level of the valve region. The ileocecal valve is clearly identifiable, as well as the different characteristics of the colonic and ileal walls on ultrasound

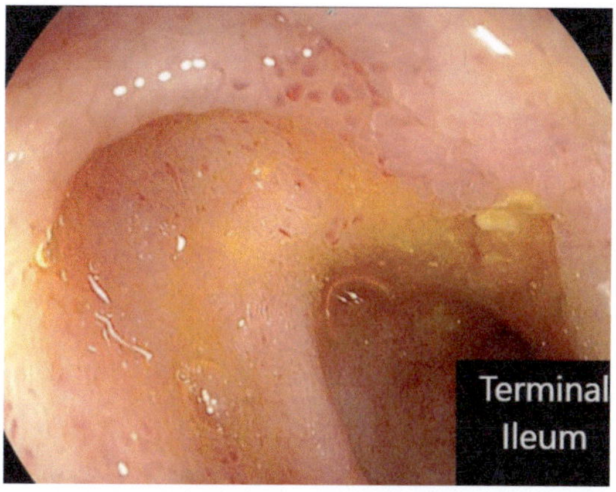

Fig. 3.26 Endoscopic view of the terminal ileum showing hyperemia without evident erosions or ulcers

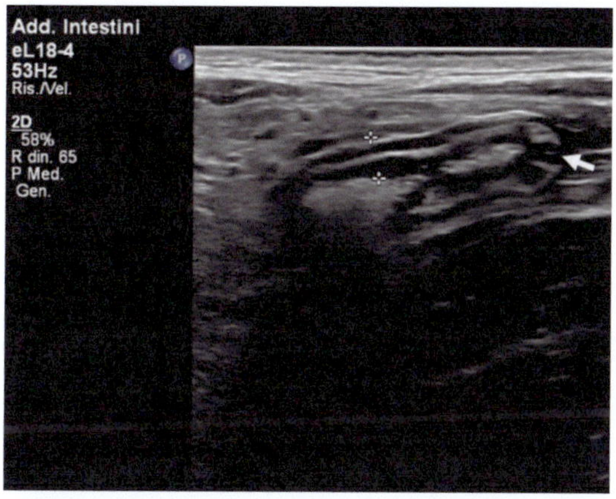

Fig. 3.27 IUS. Ileal tract with BWT up to 4.3 mm, the mucosal contour appears irregular in places, extending down to the muscular layer (white arrow). These ultrasound scars correspond to deep endoscopic ulceration

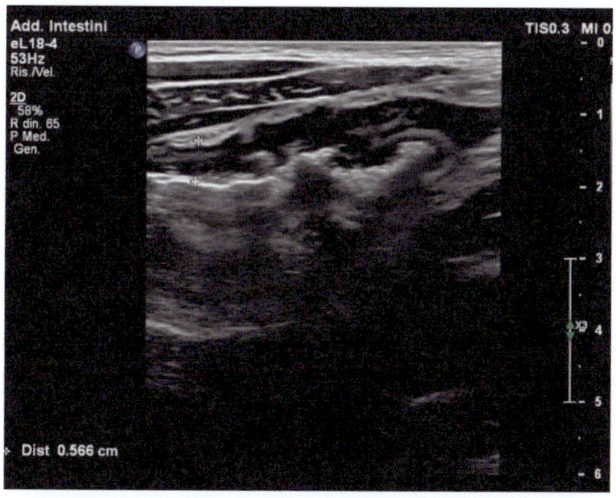

Fig. 3.28 IUS. Colonic coecum with BWT up to 5.6 mm and hypoechoic bowel wall: the mucosa profile is disrupted by the presence of some deep ulceration

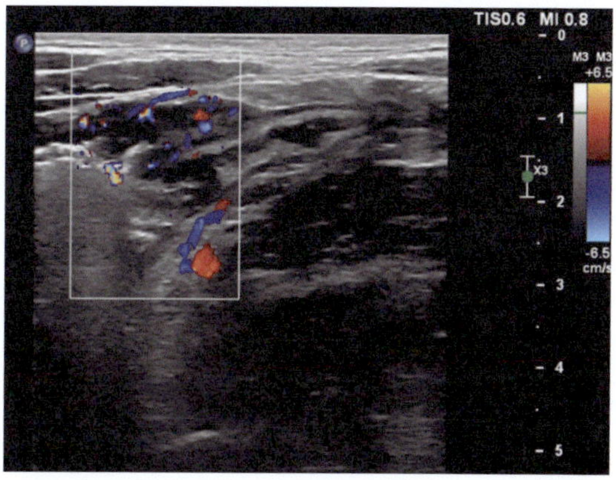

Fig. 3.29 IUS. At color Doppler analysis, increased vascularity is observed in both the bowel wall and the adjacent mesenteric fat, graded as 4 according to Limberg score

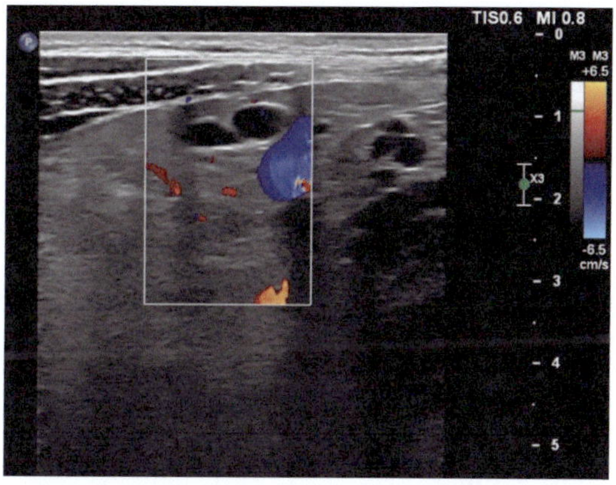

Fig. 3.30 IUS. In the mesentery surrounding the pathological bowel loop there are multiple lymph nodes with the typical ellipsoidal shape supporting the presence of an active disease

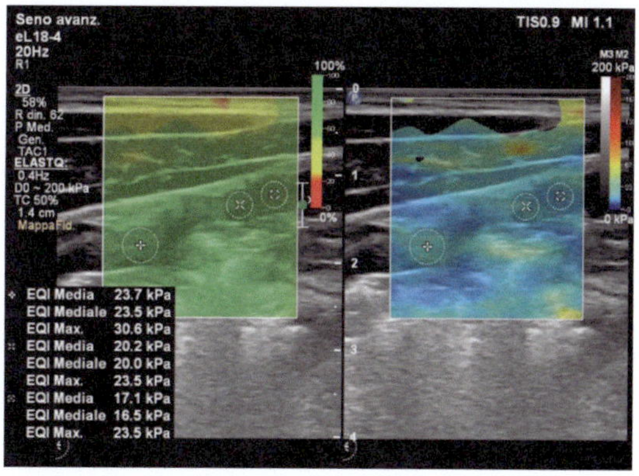

Fig. 3.31 IUS-SWE 2D shear wave elastography (2D-SWE) showing increased bowel-wall stiffness of the terminal ileum due to high-grade inflammation

3.2.6 Clinical Scenario 6: Ultrasound in Jejunal Crohn's Disease

The patient is a 28-year-old man undergoing esophagogastroduodenoscopy (EGD) for dyspepsia and vomiting, which reveals non-ulcerated duodenal erosions (Fig. 3.32).

Histology on biopsy was suggestive of IBD. Ileocolonoscopy shows no abnormalities. Small-intestine ultrasound shows hypervascularity (Fig. 3.33) and extensive thickening (Fig. 3.34) of the jejunal walls.

Small-intestine contrast ultrasonography (SICUS) highlights jejunal wall thickening (Fig. 3.35).

Video-capsule enteroscopy (VCE) reveals delayed jejunal transit, multiple substenoses (Fig. 3.36), and deep ulcers (Fig. 3.37).

3.2.7 Clinical Scenario 7: Contrast-Enhanced Ultrasound (CEUS)

A 32-year-old woman presents with abdominal pain, fever, and obstructive symptoms. A new diagnosis of Crohn's disease is suspected after an abdominal CT scan suggests terminal ileitis (Fig. 3.38). IUS reveals an ileal tract with BWT up to 9.4 mm (Figs. 3.39, 3.40, and 3.41) for a tract extending about 10 cm, loss of normal wall stratification, and enlarged lymph nodes (Fig. 3.40).

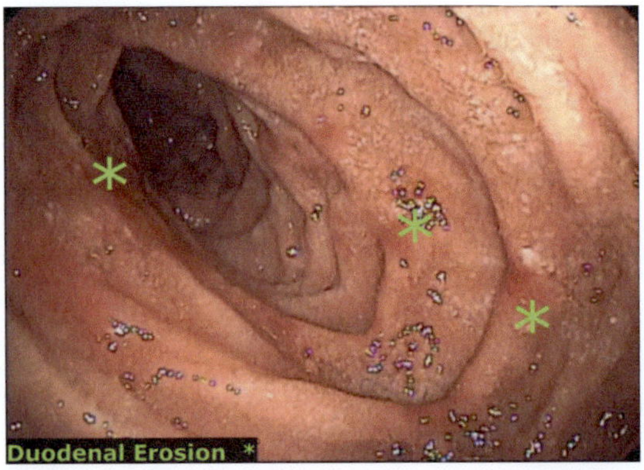

Fig. 3.32 EGD. Upper endoscopy shows small duodenal erosions

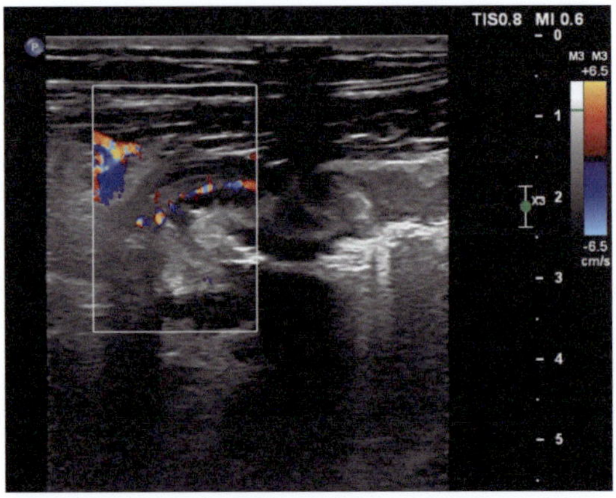

Fig. 3.33 IUS. Diffuse hypervascularization of small intestine loops in extensive Crohn's disease

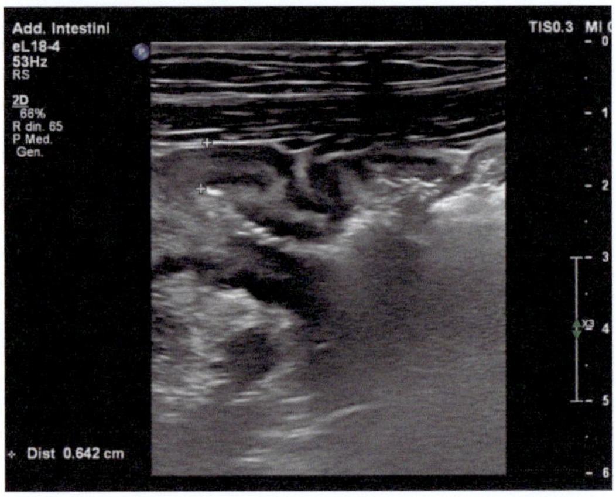

Fig. 3.34 IUS image showing a dilated small bowel loop with thickened bowel wall demonstrating plica hypertrophy. The irregular appearance of the mucosal layer is consistent with multiple deep ulceration showed at VCE

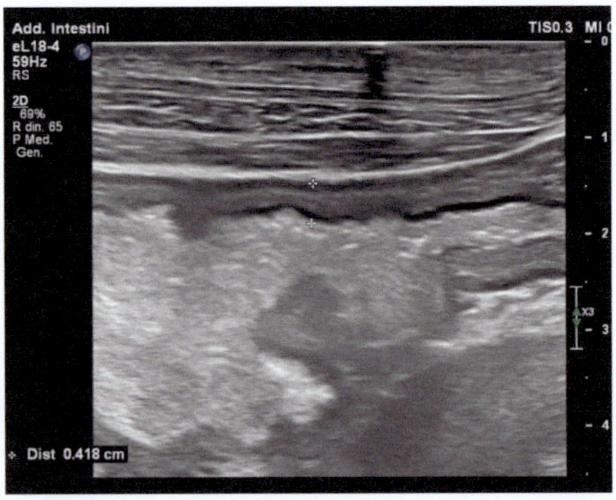

Fig. 3.35 IUS. The use of oral contrast (SICUS) enhances the ultrasound features of small intestine loops by distending them, clearly delineating their edges

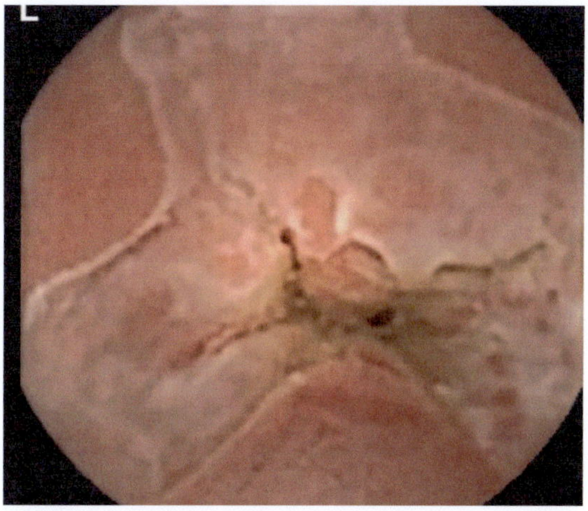

Fig. 3.36 VCE. Endoscopic view of a jejunal stricture (VCE)

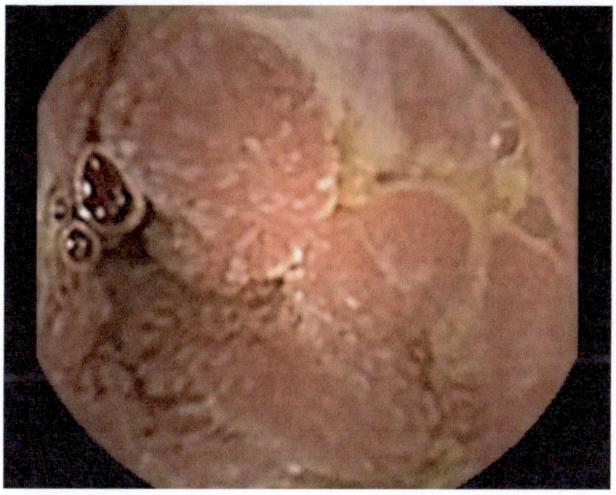

Fig. 3.37 VCE. Multiple small-bowel ulcerations

Contrast-enhanced ultrasound (CEUS) demonstrates the characteristic arterial phase contrast enhancement (Figs. 3.42, 3.43, 3.44, and 3.45) typical of moderate/severe active disease, confirmed by increased wall stiffness at SWE (Fig. 3.46).

The diagnosis of Crohn's disease with ileal involvement was confirmed and following multidisciplinary assessment ileocecal resection was performed.

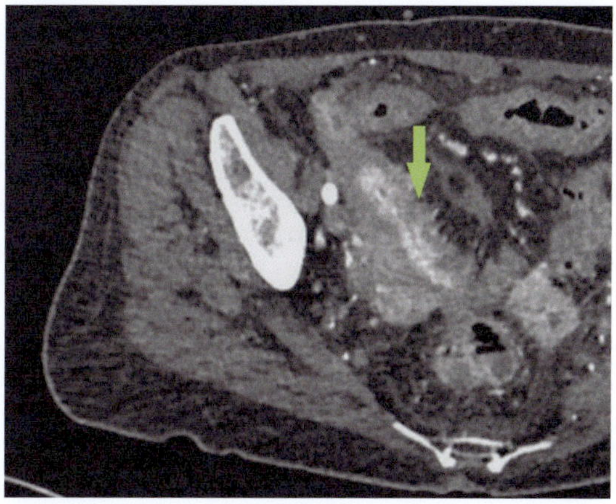

Fig. 3.38 CT scan. Prominent mesenteric vessels extending towards the affected bowel loop, giving it an appearance similar to the teeth of a comb due to a combination of vascular distension and fibrofatty proliferation of the mesentery. This is known as the "comb sign," which is specific but not pathognomonic of active Crohn's disease

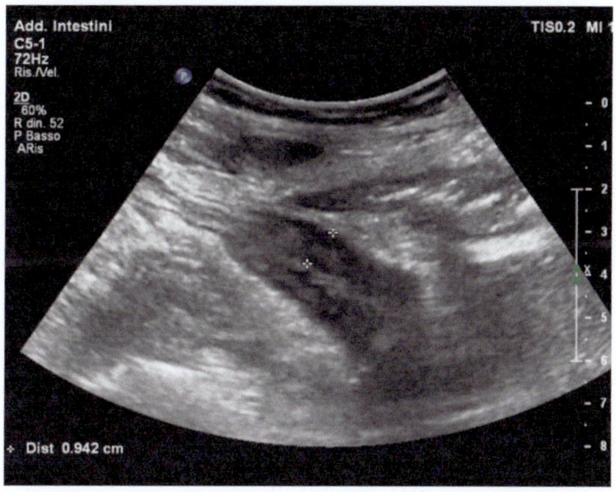

Fig. 3.39 IUS longitudinal scan with a convex probe of a thickened ileal segment with loss of wall layering

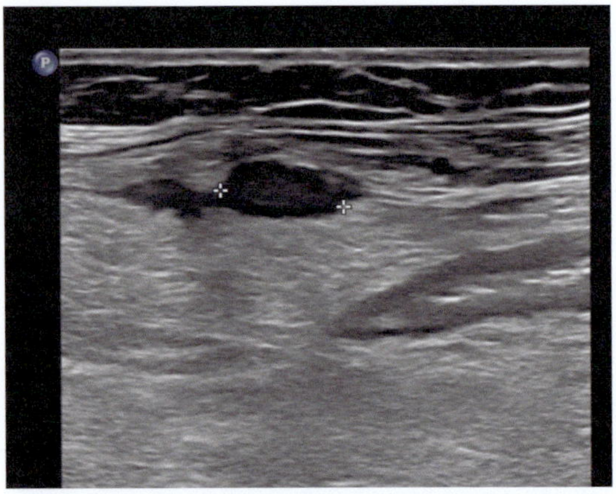

Fig. 3.40 IUS. Enlarged lymph node consistent with disease at an active phase

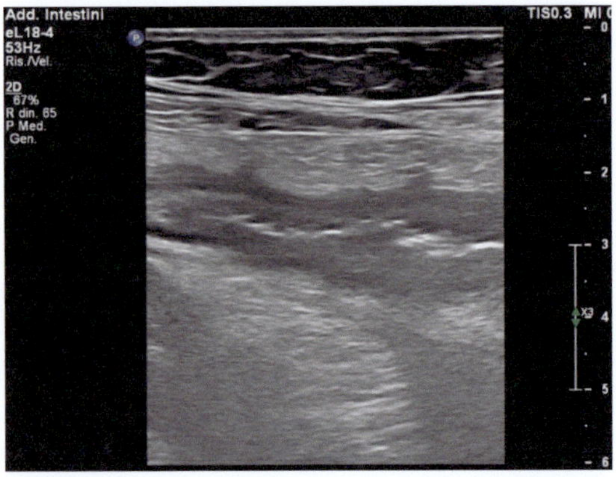

Fig. 3.41 IUS. Longitudinal scan with a high-frequency linear probe of a thickened ileal loop. The profile of the loop is irregular with small hypoechoic tracts that deepen into the adjacent hypertrophic mesentery

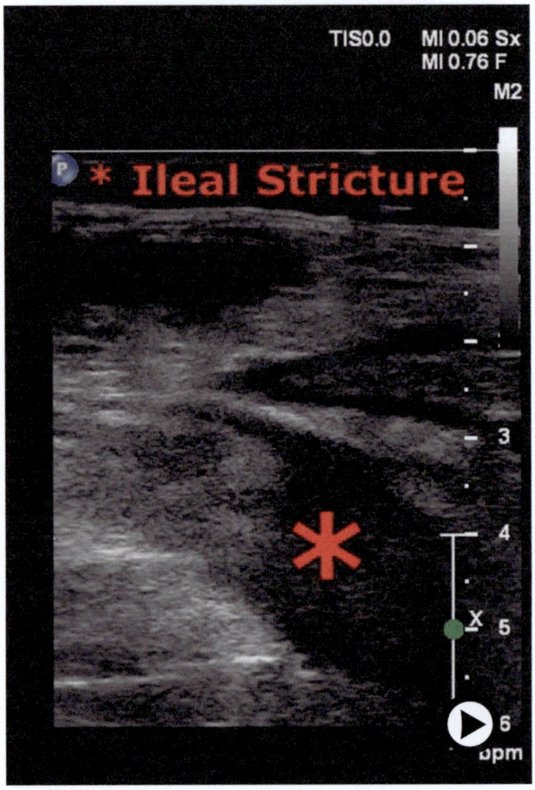

Fig. 3.42 IUS. Transverse scan of an ileal stricture (red star), the same scan will be used throughout the CEUS examination to identify contrast enhancementVideo 3.3 IUS evaluation of extensive ileal Crohn's disease and ileal CEUS (contrast-enhanced ultrasound) (▶ https://doi.org/10.1007/000-j1z)

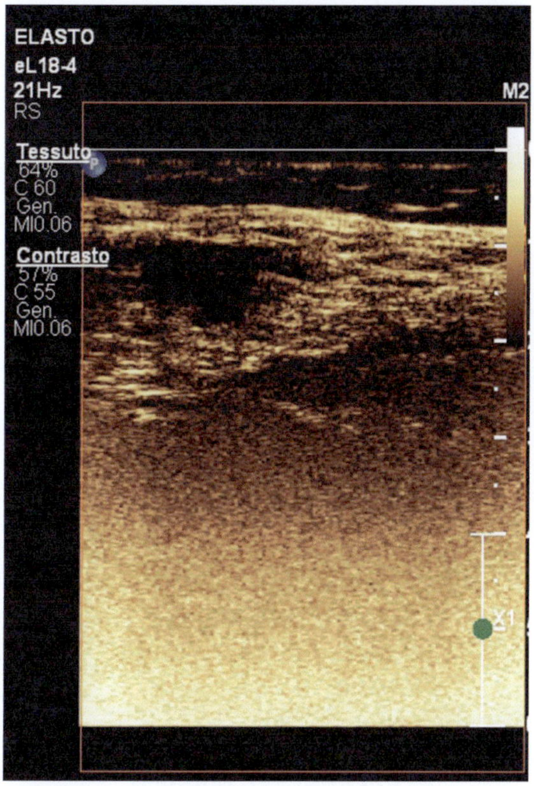

Fig. 3.43 IUS-CEUS T0: Contrast mode, prior to intravenous injection of ultrasound contrast agent (UCA) (SonoVue®). Towards the lower part of the image, ileal thickening is not distinguishable at this phase

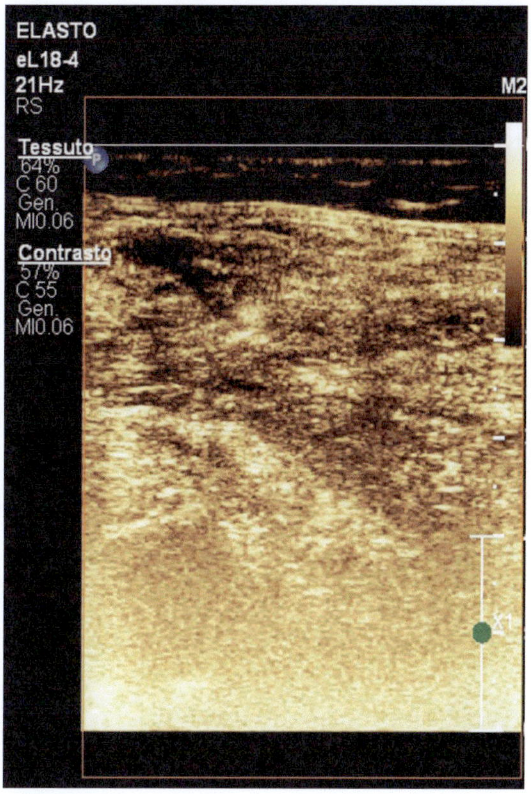

Fig. 3.44 IUS-CEUS T1: Arterial phase, 33 s from intravenous injection of UCA. Ileal BWT is clearly identifiable, contrast enhancement is concentrated in the mucosal and submucosal layer and partially in the surrounding mesenteric fat, indicative of moderate/severe disease activity

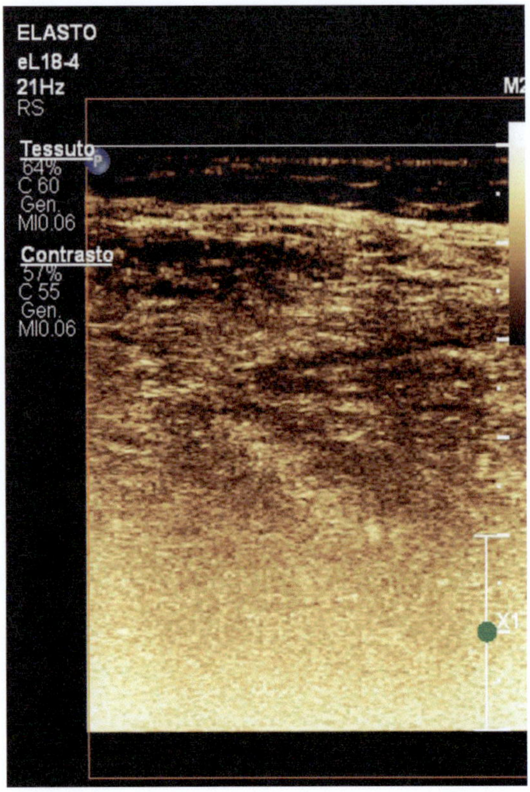

Fig. 3.45 IUS-CEUS T2: 120 s from contrast injection. The contrast media has almost all been removed from the bowel loop

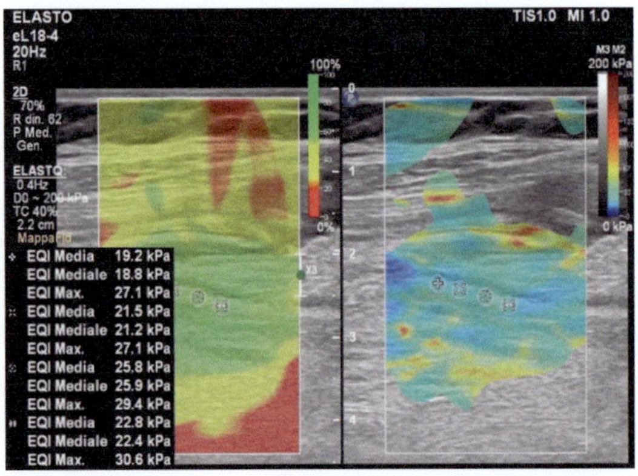

Fig. 3.46 IUS. Multi-parametric ultrasound was completed with 2D shear wave elastography (2D-SWE), which demonstrates increased stiffness, a finding compatible with the suspected disease activity

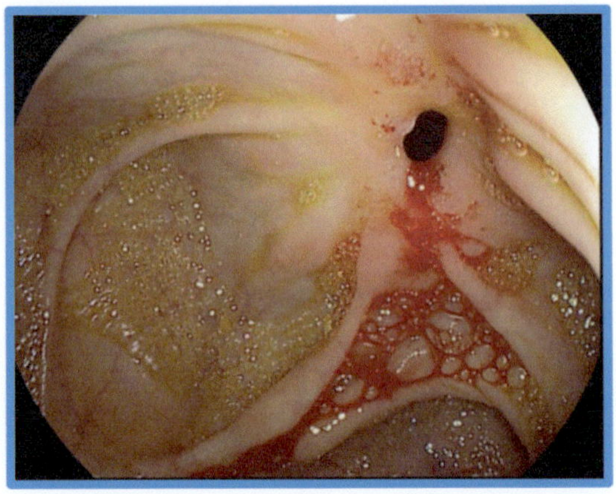

Fig. 3.47 End-to-end ileocecal anastomosis, severe anastomotic recurrence (Rutgeerts i4) can be identified by a stenosis that is non-passable by the scope

3.3 Evaluating the Response to Treatment in Crohn's Disease

3.3.1 Clinical Scenario 8: Lack of Response to Medical Therapy

A 43-year-old man with ileal Crohn's disease (A1-L1-B2 according to the Montreal classification) underwent ileocecal resection with functional end-to-end anastomosis 20 years ago. Subsequent post-operative recurrence (i3 according to Rutgeerts' criteria), demonstrated failure of the infliximab-adalimumab therapy. Due to disease progression with endoscopic Rutgeerts i4 anastomotic recurrence (Fig. 3.47), neoterminal ileum thickening (Figs. 3.48, 3.49, 3.50, 3.51, and 3.52) and hypervascularization (Limberg score type 2, Fig. 3.53), a switch to ustekinumab was made. Transmural monitoring after 1 year of treatment did not show improvement in the extension of disease (Fig. 3.52), with persisting hypervascularization of the neoterminal ileum (Fig. 3.54) with wall thickness up to 7 mm (Fig. 3.49). SWE

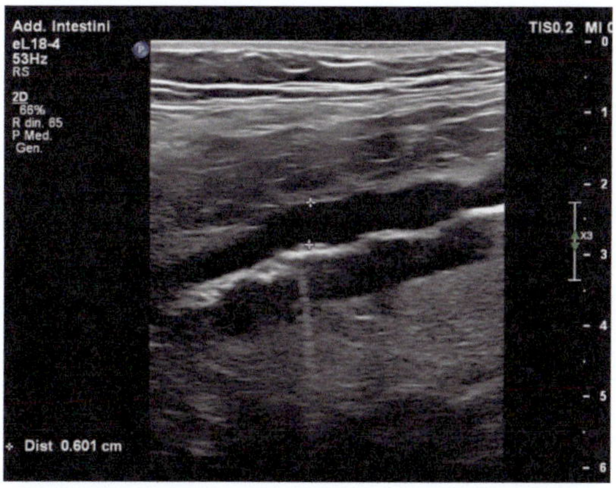

Fig. 3.48 IUS. Transverse US scan of involved ileum showing thickening up to 6 mm and complete loss of bowel-wall stratification; a hypertrophic submucosal layer can also be seen

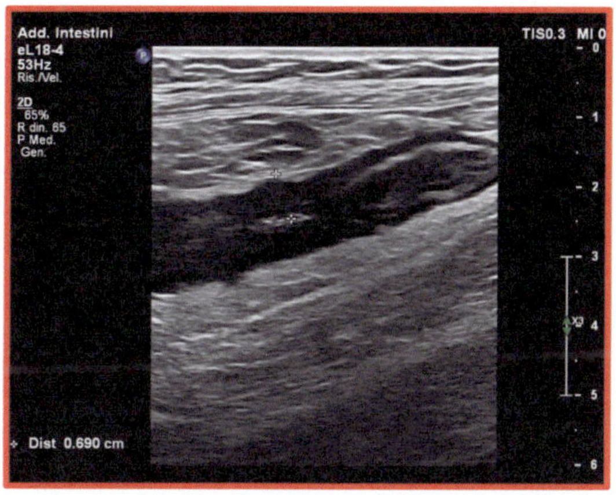

Fig. 3.49 IUS. No evidence of transmural improvement after 1 year of medical treatment should suggest an adjustment of therapeutic strategy according to a treat-to-target model

showed a lack of decrease values in bowel wall stiffness, suggesting a lack of transmural healing (Figs. 3.56 and 3.51). Endoscopic, CT, and IUS aspects of the surgical anastomosis can be seen in Figs. 3.47, 3.55, and 3.56 respectively.

Blue frame: Pre-treatment images, Red frame: Post-treatment images.

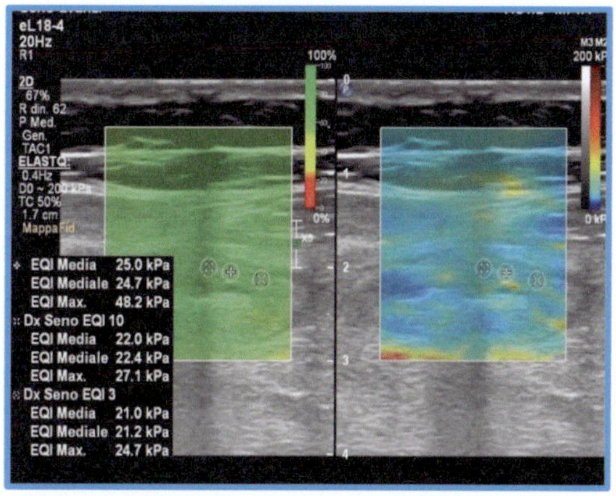

Fig. 3.50 IUS-SWE exam shows increased stiffness within the affected bowel wall up to 20–25 kPa, which, together with other activity assessment signs, suggests active disease

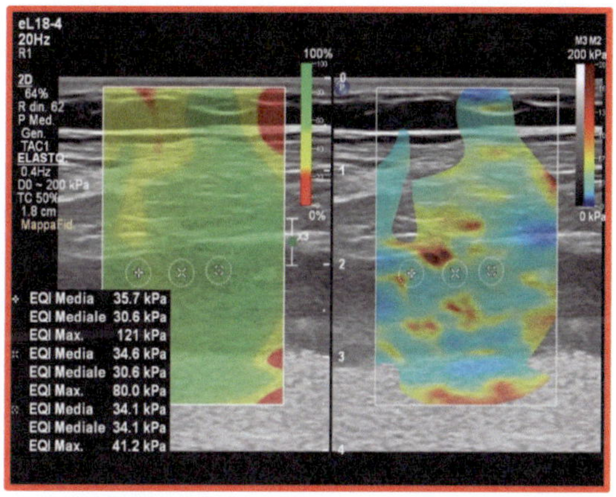

Fig. 3.51 IUS-SWE. No data are currently available on stiffness response to treatment and its interpretation. Nevertheless, the lack of decreasing values (25–35 kPa) also suggests a lack of transmural healing

3.3.2 Clinical Scenario 9: Disease Recurrence After Surgery

The patient is a 39-year-old man patient affected by severe ileal-colonic Crohn's disease not responding to multiple biological drugs (infliximab, ustekinumab, risankizumab). In 2022 he underwent ileocecal resection. In 2023 he was

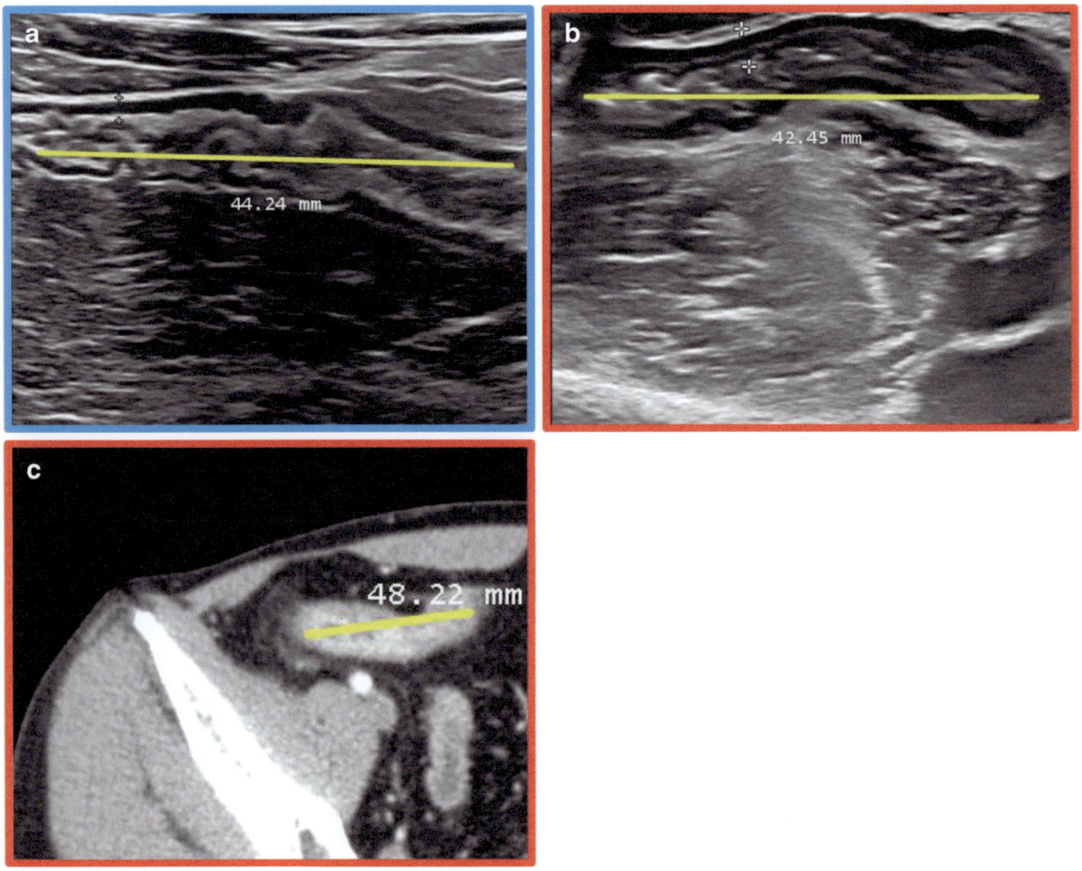

Fig. 3.52 IUS. No disease extension was observed before and after ustekinumab treatment (**a**, **b**). Interestingly, findings from US and CT enterography (**b**, **c**) demonstrate a significant agreement in defining disease extension

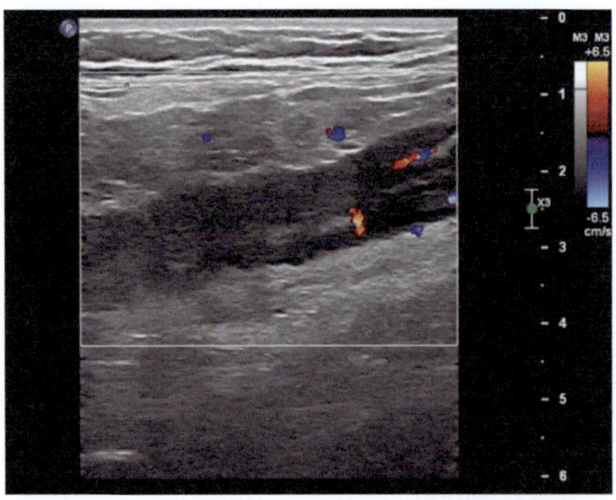

Fig. 3.53 IUS. Increased vascularity within the bowel wall of neoterminal ileum shown by color Doppler US hypervascularization (Limberg score 2)

started on Upadacitinib due to symptomatic anastomotic and colonic disease recurrence.

Colonoscopy showed Rutgeerts-i4 anastomotic recurrence with a non-passable neoterminal ileum stenosis (Fig. 3.57), deep ulcers in the anastomotic region (Fig. 3.58), and, in the right colon, the presence of deep ulcers with inflamed mucosa interposed (Fig. 3.59).

IUS shows thickened walls in the neo-ileum (Fig. 3.60) and right colon (Figs. 3.61, 3.62, and 3.63), with mesenteric and bowel wall hypervascularity (Fig. 3.62), and lymphadenopathy (Fig. 3.64).

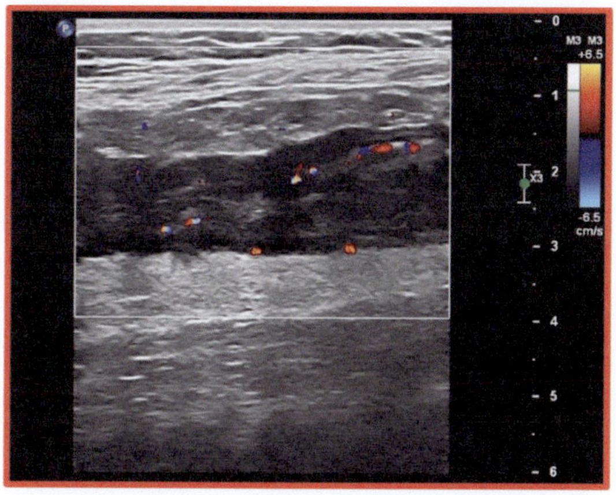

Fig. 3.54 IUS. Persisting increased blood flow in the neoterminal ileum is a sign of active disease, suggesting the absence of response after 1 year of treatment

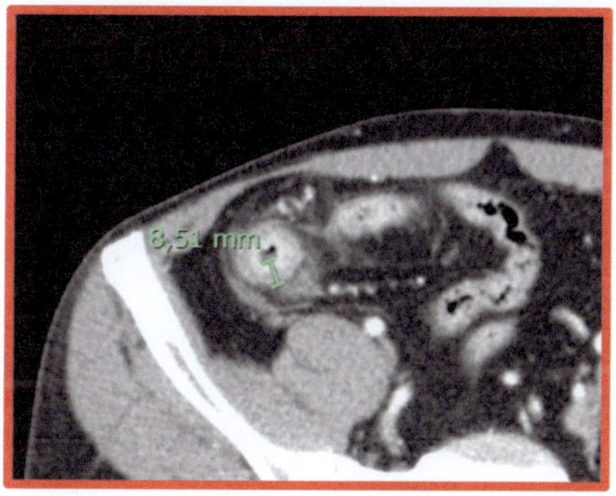

Fig. 3.55 CT enterography, "target sign" in cross-section: bright ring of mucosal enhancement, indicating severe inflammation

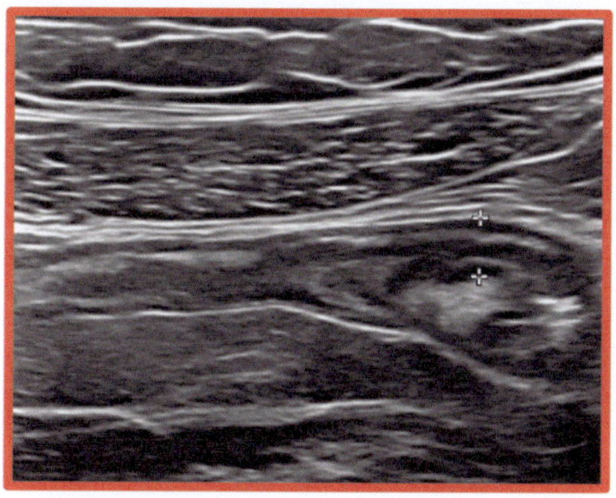

Fig. 3.56 IUS. Ileocecal region with BWT

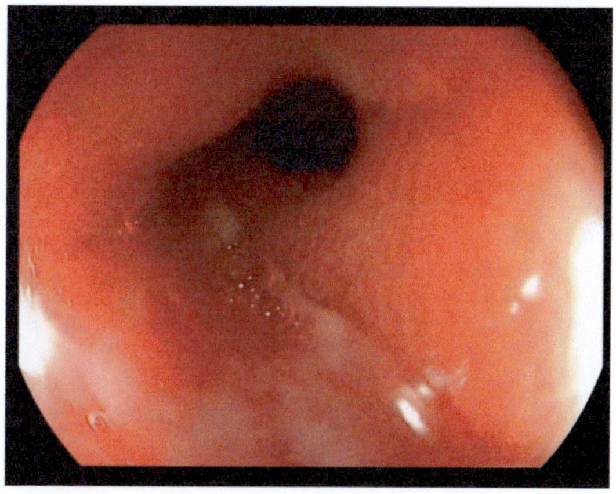

Fig. 3.57 Endoscopy. Stenosis of the ileo-colonic anastomosis, non-passable by the scope (Rutgeerts i4). Two ulcers can be seen on the edge of the stenosis

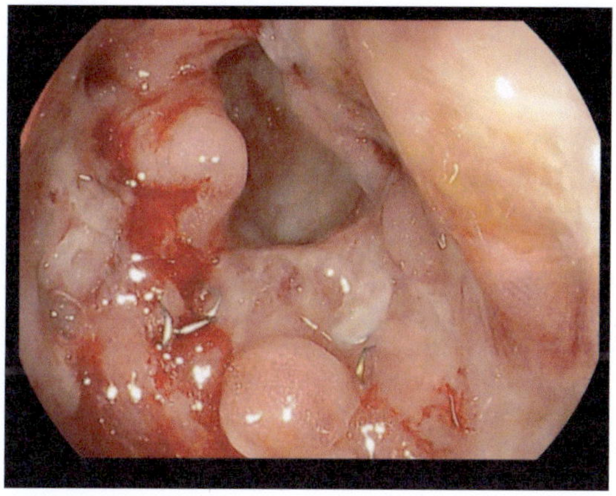

Fig. 3.58 Endoscopy. The anastomotic region can be identified by the presence of surgical clips. Deep ulcers and inflammatory pseudopolyps are present circumferentially

3.3.3 Clinical Scenario 10: Response to Medical Therapy

The patient is a 46-year-old woman with an ileocecal Crohn's disease (A2-L3-B3p). Anti-TNF therapy with adalimumab was started. Due to penetrating disease ileocecal resection and two ileal resections were performed during the disease history.

IUS was performed for a sub-occlusive episode revealing an anastomotic stricture.

A scan performed with a high-frequency, linear probe, passing through the anastomotic region characterized a stenotic lumen with hyper-

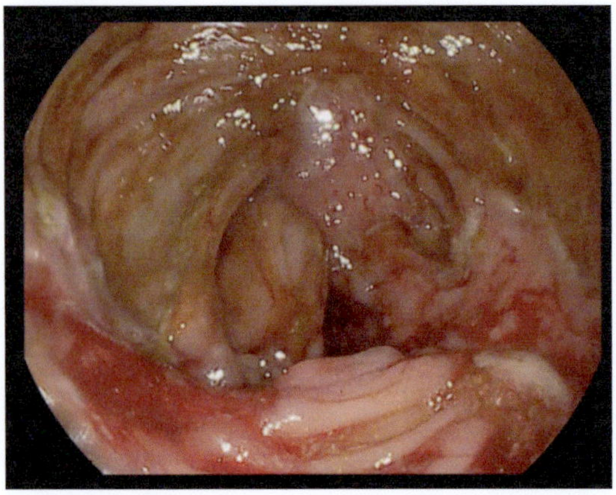

Fig. 3.59 Endoscopy. The disease has also relapsed in the right colon. Features of active disease can be seen, e.g., deep ulcers and areas of inflamed interposed mucosa

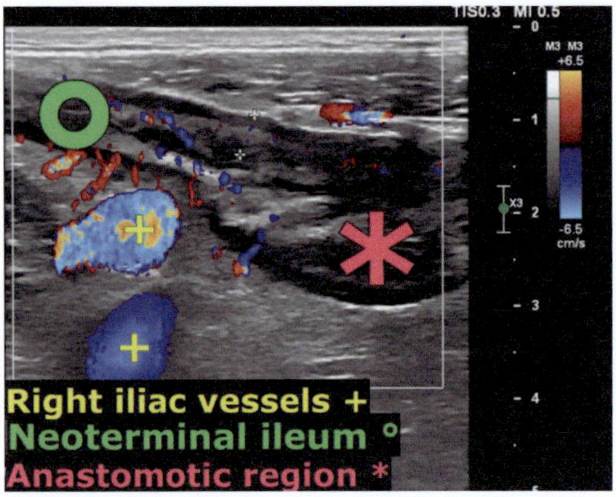

Fig. 3.60 IUS. Anastomotic region in transverse scan. Right ileal vessels are important reference points for the precise recognition of neoterminal ileum (°) and anastomotic region (*). Diffuse increased blood flow at CD and ileal BWT up to 0.55 mm are significant features for anastomotic recurrence of Crohn's disease

vascularity (Fig. 3.67). Another scan passing for the right iliac fossa conducted with a low-frequency convex probe showed a marked pre-stenotic dilatation (Fig. 3.68). The endoscopic evaluation at baseline showed an anastomotic recurrence i3 according to the Rutgeerts score and deep ulcers in the pre-anastomotic ileum (Figs. 3.69 and 3.70).

The patient started on risankizumab, obtaining an endoscopic response (Figs. 3.71 and 3.72) and despite incomplete mucosal healing and partial

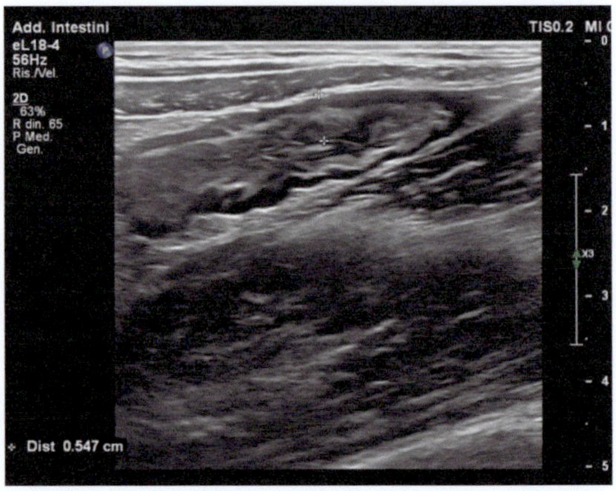

Fig. 3.61 IUS. Right colon with BWT up to 5.4 mm, with maintained bowel wall stratification

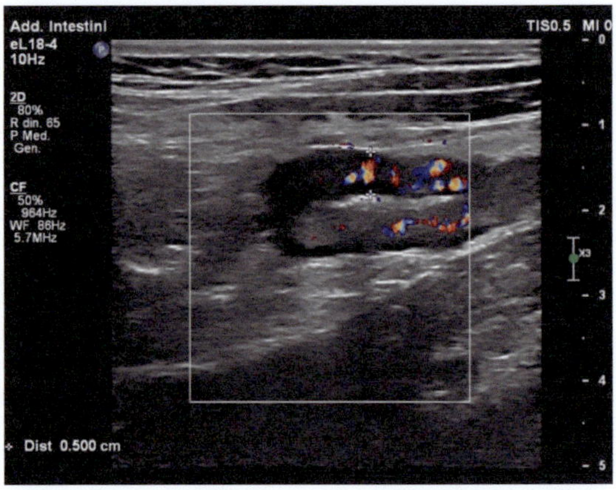

Fig. 3.62 IUS. Transverse scan of the neo terminal ileum demonstrating increased vascularization within the bowel wall at CD analysis

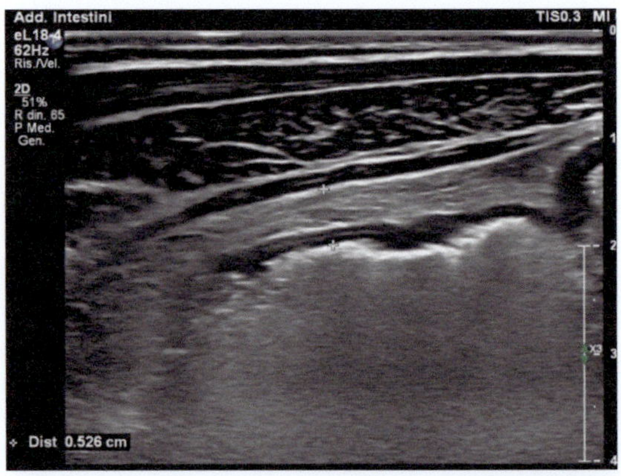

Fig. 3.63 IUS. Longitudinal scan of right colon with BWT up to 5 mm. A submucosal layer hypertrophy can be noted

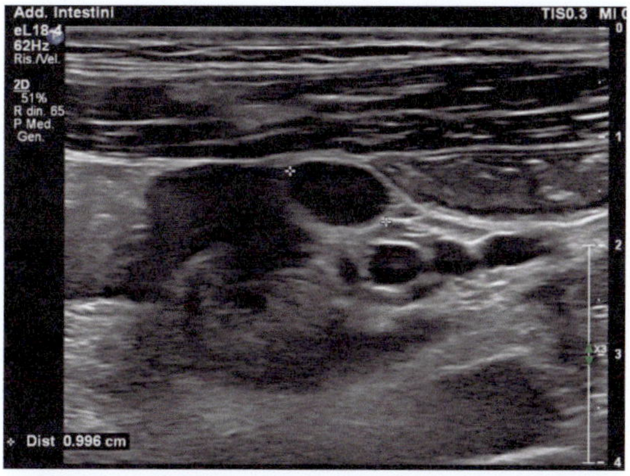

Fig. 3.64 IUS. Reactive enlarged mesenteric lymph node with typical US features: homogeneously hypoechoic oval-shaped nodule surrounded by regular borders

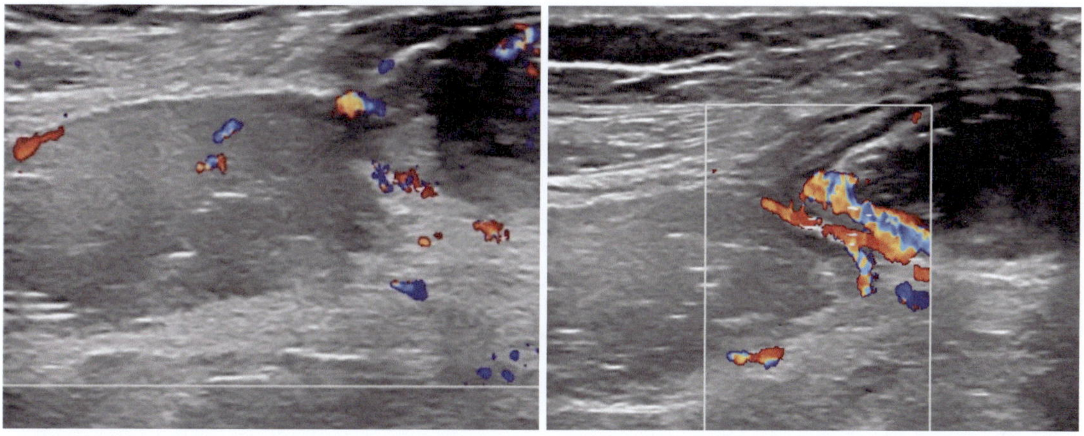

Figs. 3.65 and 3.66 IUS scans passing through the anastomotic region highlight selective hypervascularization of the surgical anastomosis

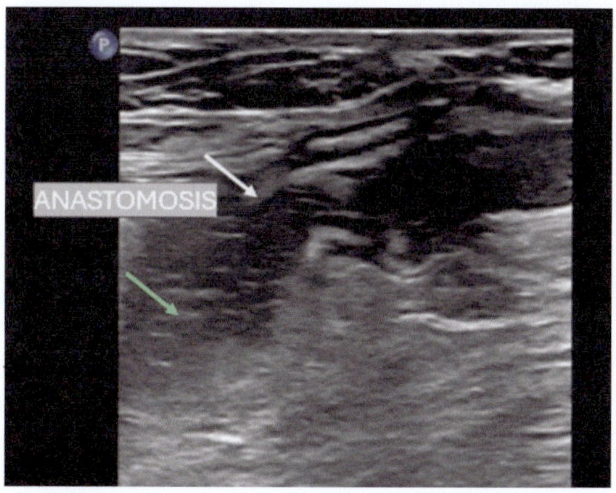

Fig. 3.67 IUS. Longitudinal scan by a high-frequency linear probe passing through the anastomotic region. A stenotic anastomotic area (white arrow) can be noted with a pre-stenotic dilatation (green arrow)

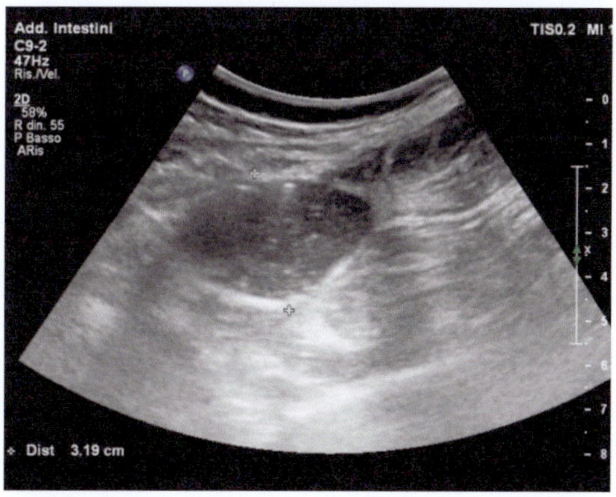

Fig. 3.68 IUS. Pre-stenotic dilation upstream of the anastomotic stenosis, the loop is dilated to approximately 3 cm and filled with enteric material

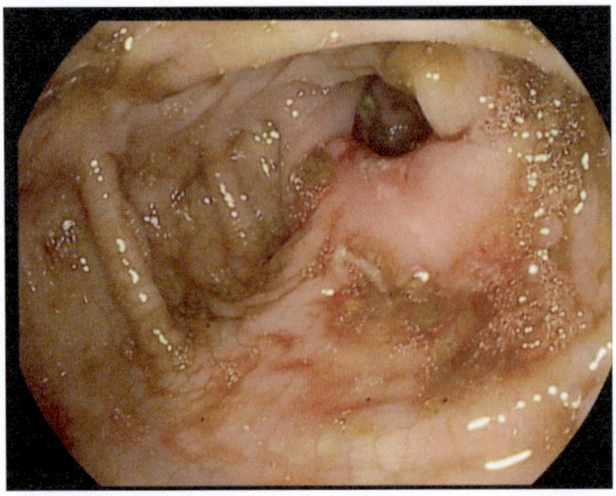

Fig. 3.69 Endoscopy. Recurrence of Crohn's disease at the anastomosis compatible with Rutgeerts score i3

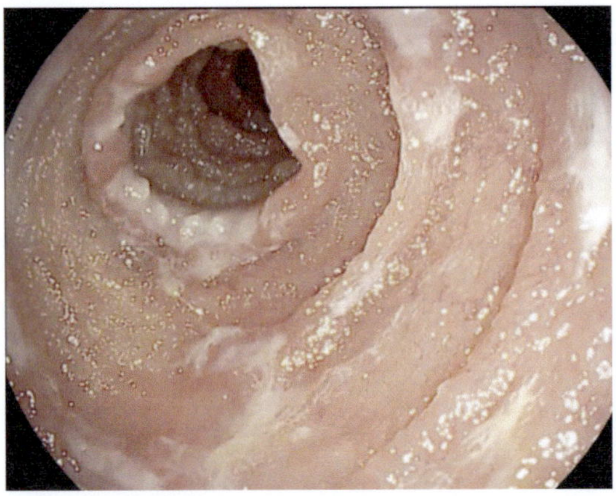

Fig. 3.70 Endoscopy. Diffuse ulcerations in pre-anastomotic ileum

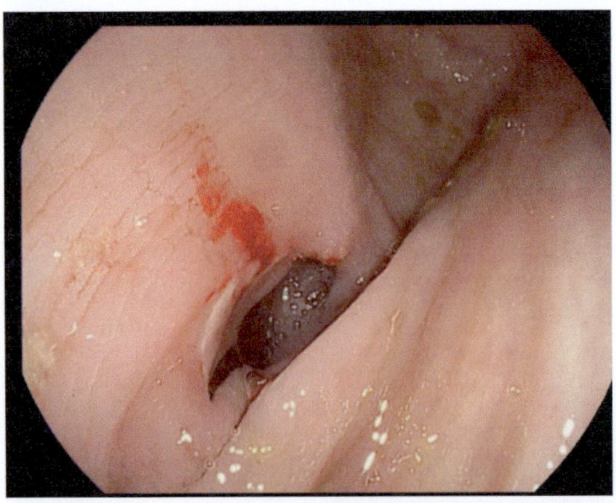

Fig. 3.71 Endoscopic view of the anastomosis from the colon; when compared with pre-treatment imaging, it can be defined as endoscopic response

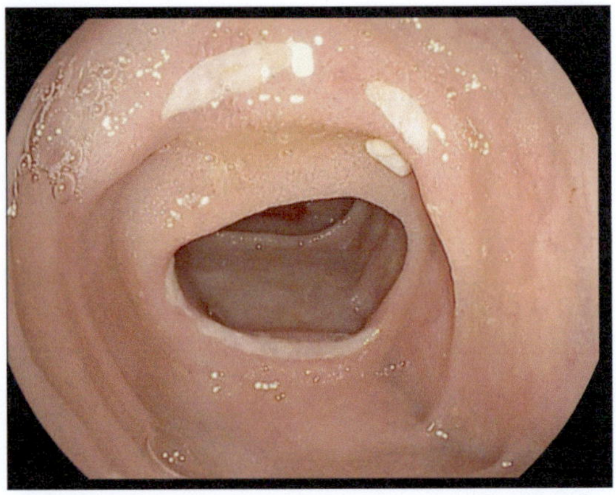

Fig. 3.72 Endoscopic view of the pre-anastomotic ileum: some ulcers persist

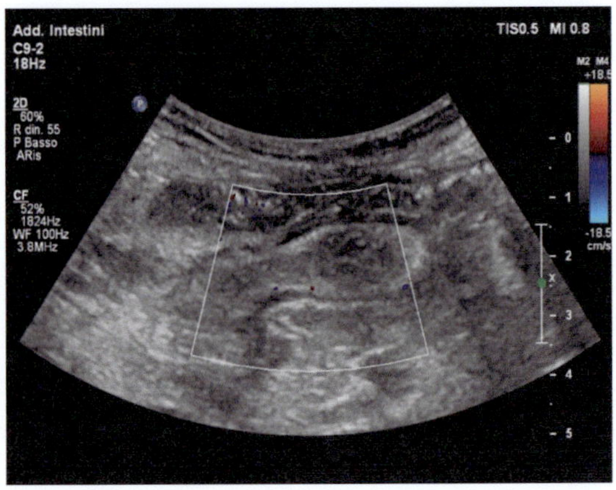

Fig. 3.73 IUS. The anastomotic region still presents BWT. However, in the absence of vascularization at follow-up with CD, this suggests a possible fibrotic evolution of the thickening

transmural response, with persisting thickening in the anastomotic region (Fig. 3.73) but with decreased vascular signal on ECD, persisting detectable only on micro-power Doppler (CPA) (Fig. 3.74).

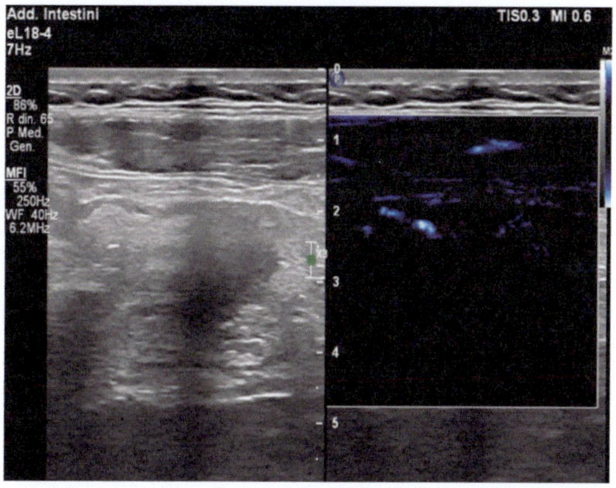

Fig. 3.74 IUS. Minimal vascular signals in the valvular region can be visualized using micro CPA Doppler modality

References

1. Maconi G, Nylund K, Ripolles T, Calabrese E, Dirks K, Dietrich CF, Hollerweger A, Sporea I, Saftoiu A, Maaser C, Hausken T, Higginson AP, Nürnberg D, Pallotta N, Romanini L, Serra C, Gilja OH. EFSUMB recommendations and clinical guidelines for intestinal ultrasound (GIUS) in inflammatory bowel diseases. Ultraschall Med. 2018;39:304–17.
2. Dolinger MT, Kayal M. Intestinal ultrasound as a non-invasive tool to monitor inflammatory bowel disease activity and guide clinical decision making. World J Gastroenterol. 2023;29(15):2272–82. https://doi.org/10.3748/wjg.v29.i15.2272. PMID: 37124889; PMCID: PMC10134421.
3. Rimola J, Torres J, Kumar S, Taylor SA, Kucharzik T. Recent advances in clinical practice: advances in cross-sectional imaging in inflammatory bowel disease. Gut. 2022;71(12):2587–97. https://doi.org/10.1136/gutjnl-2021-326562. Epub 2022 Aug 4. PMID: 35927032; PMCID: PMC9664122.
4. Yuksel I, Kilincalp S, Coskun Y, Akinci H, Hamamci M, Alkan A. Diagnostic accuracy of intestinal ultrasound and magnetic resonance enterography for the detection of endoscopy-based disease activity in ileocolonic Crohn's disease. Eur J Gastroenterol Hepatol. 2019;31(7):809–16. https://doi.org/10.1097/MEG.0000000000001438. PMID: 31094855.
5. Dragoni G, Gottin M, Innocenti T, Lynch EN, Bagnoli S, Macrì G, Bonanomi AG, Orlandini B, Rogai F, Milani S, Galli A, Milla M, Biagini MR. Correlation of ultrasound scores with endoscopic activity in Crohn's disease: a prospective exploratory study. J Crohns Colitis. 2023;17(9):1387–94. https://doi.org/10.1093/ecco-jcc/jjad068. PMID: 37023010.
6. Fraquelli M, Colli A, Casazza G, Paggi S, Colucci A, Massironi S, Duca P, Conte D. Role of US in detection of Crohn disease: meta-analysis. Radiology. 2005;236(1):95–101. https://doi.org/10.1148/radiol.2361040799. PMID: 15987966.
7. Dong J, Wang H, Zhao J, Zhu W, Zhang L, Gong J, Li Y, Gu L, Li J. Ultrasound as a diagnostic tool in detecting active Crohn's disease: a meta-analysis of prospective studies. Eur Radiol. 2014;24(1):26–33. https://doi.org/10.1007/s00330-013-2973-0. Epub 2013 Aug 7. PMID: 23921767.
8. Alkim C, Alkim H, Koksal AR, Boga S, Sen I. Angiogenesis in inflammatory bowel disease. Int J Inflam. 2015;2015:970890. https://doi.org/10.1155/2015/970890. Epub 2015 Dec 29. PMID: 26839731; PMCID: PMC4709626.
9. Furfaro F, Dal Buono A, Allocca M, D'Amico F, Zilli A, Gabbiadini R, Danese S. Bowel ultrasound in inflammatory bowel disease: how far in the grayscale? Life (Basel). 2021;11(7):649. https://doi.org/10.3390/life11070649. PMID: 34357022; PMCID: PMC8308056.
10. Sasaki T, Kunisaki R, Kinoshita H, Kimura H, Kodera T, Nozawa A, Hanzawa A, Shibata N, Yonezawa H, Miyajima E, Morita S, Fujii S, Numata K, Tanaka K, Tanaka M, Maeda S. Doppler ultrasound findings correlate with tissue vascularity and inflammation in surgical pathology specimens from patients with small intestinal Crohn's disease. BMC Res Notes. 2014;7:363. https://doi.org/10.1186/1756-0500-7-363. PMID: 24927748; PMCID: PMC4080771.
11. Paredes JM, Ripollés T, Algarra Á, Diaz R, Moreno N, Latorre P, Martínez MJ, Llopis P, López A, Moreno-Osset E. Intestinal ultrasonography and fecal calprotectin for monitoring inflammation of ileal Crohn's disease: two complementary tests. Intest Res. 2022;20(3):361–9. https://doi.org/10.5217/ir.2021.00126. Epub 2022 Mar 15. PMID: 35279969; PMCID: PMC9344237.
12. de Voogd F, Bots S, Gecse K, Gilja OH, D'Haens G, Nylund K. Intestinal ultrasound early on in treatment follow-up predicts endoscopic response to anti-TNFα treatment in Crohn's disease. J Crohns Colitis. 2022;16(10):1598–608. https://doi.org/10.1093/ecco-jcc/jjac072. PMID: 35639823; PMCID: PMC9624292.
13. Allocca M, Dell'Avalle C, Zilli A, Furfaro F, D'Amico F, Jairath V, Rubin DT, Peyrin-Biroulet L, Fiorino G, Danese S. Ultrasound remission after biologic induction and long-term endoscopic remission in Crohn's disease: a prospective cohort study. EClinicalMedicine. 2024;71:102559. https://doi.org/10.1016/j.eclinm.2024.102559. PMID: 38549587; PMCID: PMC10972812.
14. Sævik F, Eriksen R, Eide GE, Gilja OH, Nylund K. Development and validation of a simple ultrasound activity score for Crohn's disease. J Crohns Colitis. 2021;15(1):115–24. https://doi.org/10.1093/ecco-jcc/jjaa112. PMID: 32504533; PMCID: PMC7805799.
15. Ripollés T, Poza J, Suarez Ferrer C, Martínez-Pérez MJ, Martín-Algíbez A, de Las Heras Paez B. Evaluation of Crohn's disease activity: develop-

ment of an ultrasound score in a multicenter study. Inflamm Bowel Dis. 2021;27(1):145–54. https://doi.org/10.1093/ibd/izaa134. PMID: 32507880.

16. Maconi G, Carsana L, Fociani P, Sampietro GM, Ardizzone S, Cristaldi M, Parente F, Vago GL, Taschieri AM, Bianchi Porro G. Small bowel stenosis in Crohn's disease: clinical, biochemical and ultrasonographic evaluation of histological features. Aliment Pharmacol Ther. 2003;18(7):749–56. https://doi.org/10.1046/j.1365-2036.2003.01673.x. PMID: 14510749.
17. Ripollés T, Martínez-Pérez MJ, Blanc E, Delgado F, Vizuete J, Paredes JM, Vilar J. Contrast-enhanced ultrasound (CEUS) in Crohn's disease: technique, image interpretation and clinical applications. Insights Imaging. 2011;2(6):639–52. https://doi.org/10.1007/s13244-011-0124-1. Epub 2011 Aug 10. PMID: 22347983; PMCID: PMC3259412.
18. Medellin A, Merrill C, Wilson SR. Role of contrast-enhanced ultrasound in evaluation of the bowel. Abdom Radiol (NY). 2018;43(4):918–33. https://doi.org/10.1007/s00261-017-1399-6. PMID: 29260278; PMCID: PMC5884905.
19. De Franco A, Di Veronica A, Armuzzi A, Roberto I, Marzo M, De Pascalis B, De Vitis I, Papa A, Bock E, Danza FM, Bonomo L, Guidi L. Ileal Crohn disease: mural microvascularity quantified with contrast-enhanced US correlates with disease activity. Radiology. 2012;262(2):680–8. https://doi.org/10.1148/radiol.11110440. Epub 2011 Dec 12. PMID: 22157203.
20. Migaleddu V, Scanu AM, Quaia E, Rocca PC, Dore MP, Scanu D, Azzali L, Virgilio G. Contrast-enhanced ultrasonographic evaluation of inflammatory activity in Crohn's disease. Gastroenterology. 2009;137(1):43–52. https://doi.org/10.1053/j.gastro.2009.03.062. Epub 2009 May 5. PMID: 19422826.
21. Quaia E, Migaleddu V, Baratella E, Pizzolato R, Rossi A, Grotto M, Cova MA. The diagnostic value of small bowel wall vascularity after sulfur hexafluoride-filled microbubble injection in patients with Crohn's disease. Correlation with the therapeutic effectiveness of specific anti-inflammatory treatment. Eur J Radiol. 2009;69(3):438–44. https://doi.org/10.1016/j.ejrad.2008.10.029. Epub 2008 Dec 12. PMID: 19070446.
22. Serafin Z, Białecki M, Białecka A, Sconfienza LM, Kłopocka M. Contrast-enhanced ultrasound for detection of Crohn's disease activity: systematic review and meta-analysis. J Crohns Colitis. 2016;10(3):354–62. https://doi.org/10.1093/ecco-jcc/jjv196. Epub 2015 Oct 27. PMID: 26507861; PMCID: PMC4957465.
23. Liu C, Xu XR, Xu HX, Liu ZJ, Zhang YF, Sun LP, Xu JM, Liu LN, Guo LH, Bo XW. Conventional ultrasound and contrast-enhanced ultrasound in evaluating the severity of Crohn's disease. Int J Clin Exp Med. 2015;8(1):123–34. PMID: 25784981; PMCID: PMC4358436.
24. Ma X, Li Y, Jia H, Zhang J, Wang G, Liu X, Song Y. Contrast-enhanced ultrasound in the diagnosis of patients suspected of having active Crohn's disease: meta-analysis. Ultrasound Med Biol. 2015;41(3):659–68. https://doi.org/10.1016/j.ultrasmedbio.2014.09.013. Epub 2015 Jan 22. PMID: 25619783.
25. Ripollés T, Rausell N, Paredes JM, Grau E, Martínez MJ, Vizuete J. Effectiveness of contrast-enhanced ultrasound for characterisation of intestinal inflammation in Crohn's disease: a comparison with surgical histopathology analysis. J Crohns Colitis. 2013;7(2):120–8. https://doi.org/10.1016/j.crohns.2012.03.002. Epub 2012 Apr 5. PMID: 22483566.
26. Limberg B. Diagnosis of chronic inflammatory bowel disease by ultrasonography. Z Gastroenterol. 1999;37:495–508.
27. Novak KL, Nylund K, Maaser C, Petersen F, Kucharzik T, Lu C, Allocca M, Maconi G, de Voogd F, Christensen B, Vaughan R, Palmela C, Carter D, Wilkens R. Expert Consensus on Optimal Acquisition and Development of the International Bowel Ultrasound Segmental Activity Score [IBUS-SAS]: a reliability and inter-rater variability study on intestinal ultrasonography in Crohn's disease. J Crohns Colitis. 2021;15(4):609–16. https://doi.org/10.1093/ecco-jcc/jjaa216. PMID: 33098642; PMCID: PMC8023841.

4 Ultrasound in Complicated Crohn's Disease: Stenosis, Fistula and Abscess

Anna Testa, Fabiana Castiglione, and Antonio Rispo

4.1 Stenosis

Patients affected by Crohn's disease (CD) can develop small bowel and, less commonly, colonic stenosis. Their prevalence increases over the course of the disease [1]. Stenosis usually cause obstructive symptoms, thus representing the main cause of surgical intervention (70–90%) [2], even if up to 20% of subjects may be asymptomatic [3]. In this setting, early recognition of this kind of complication is critical in CD management (medical vs surgical approach).

Intestinal ultrasound (IUS) is a valid tool to identify these complications in a non-invasive way. The main IUS diagnostic criteria for the detection of stenosis are: thickened and stiff bowel wall (Fig. 4.1a, b), narrowing of the lumen (diameter less than 1 cm) (Fig. 4.2, Video 4.1), proximal dilatation (>25–30 mm) (Figs. 4.3 and 4.4; Fig. 4.5, Video 4.2) and hyperperistalsis of the pre-stenotic gut [4, 5] (Fig. 4.6, Video 4.3). Sometimes, we can identify hydro-aerial levels in the dilated segment (Fig. 4.7, Video 4.4)

According to Pruijt et al., IUS's pooled sensitivity and specificity are 81 and 90%, even if not all the papers evaluated surgery as a reference standard [6].

The ingestion of polyethylene glycol (PEG) solution (500–800 mL) drunk approximately 30 min before IUS (*small intestine contrast US; SICUS*) has been shown to improve the sensitivity of IUS in patients with at least one stenosis (74% vs. 89–98%) and those with two or more strictures (55% vs. 75–77%), with an overall specificity >93% [7, 8]. Oral contrast offers more marked dilation of the pre-stenotic tract, thus allowing a better visualization of the narrowed segment. Moreover, SICUS is highly accurate in identifying pre-stenotic dilation, even with higher sensitivity than magnetic resonance enterography (MRE) [9, 10]. SICUS's pooled sensitivity and specificity in the diagnosis of stenosis are 94 and 95% [6].

Many studies have evaluated the concordance of IUS with other radiologic techniques, such as computed tomography enteroclysis and magnetic resonance enterography (MRE) [10–12]. The results of our study [12] exhibited fair concordance ($k = 0.082$; $p = 0.01$) between those two techniques in the detection of small bowel stenoses. Kumar et al. performed a comparison between SICUS and MRE and observed a sensi-

Supplementary Information The online version contains supplementary material available at https://doi.org/10.1007/978-3-032-11418-1_4. The videos can be accessed individually by clicking the DOI link in the accompanying figure caption or by scanning this link with the SN More Media App.

A. Testa (✉) · F. Castiglione · A. Rispo
Gastroenterology Unit, Department of Clinical Medicine and Surgery, University of Naples Federico II, Naples, Italy

F. Terracciano et al. (eds.), *Bowel Ultrasound Compared with Endoscopy*,
https://doi.org/10.1007/978-3-032-11418-1_4

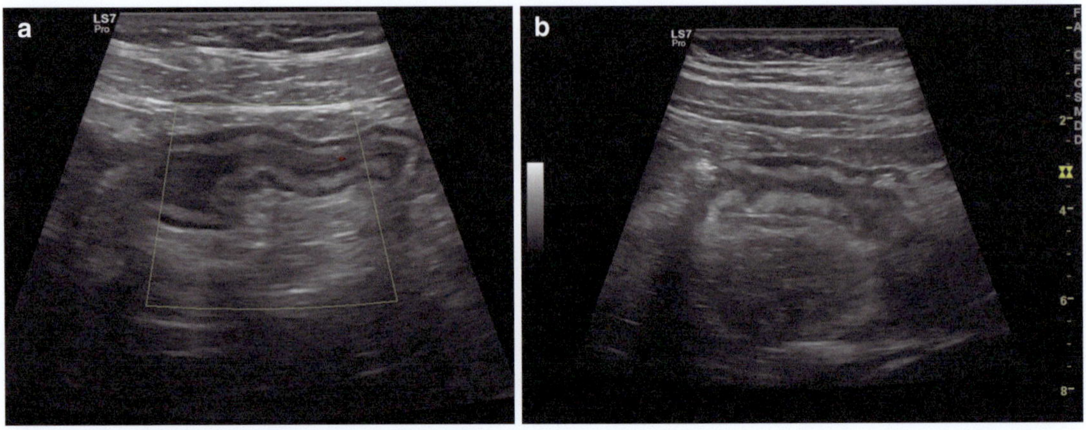

Fig. 4.1 Longitudinal image ultrasound of increased bowel wall thickness

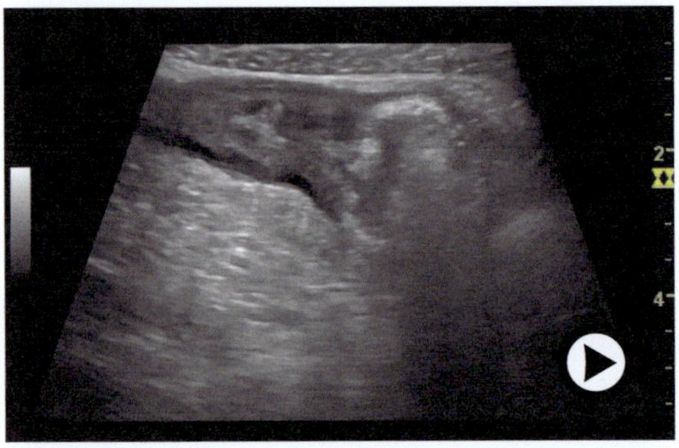

Fig. 4.2 Narrowing of the lumen identified one parameter of the stenosis (▶ https://doi.org/10.1007/000-j25)

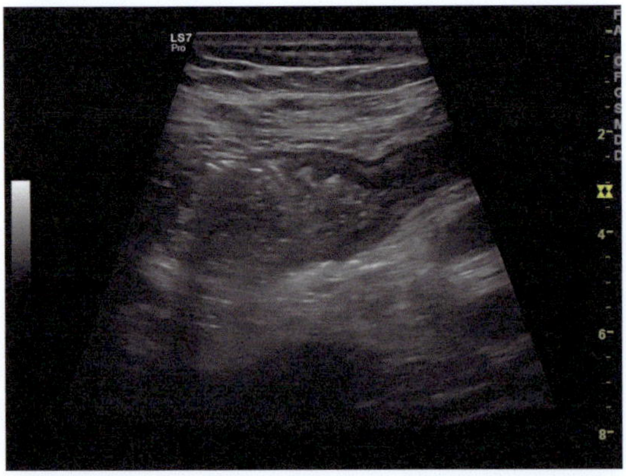

Fig. 4.3 Narrowing of lumen on intestinal ultrasound and proximal dilatation

tivity of 87.5 and 100%, respectively, for the detection of stenosis.

Stenoses in patients with CD are often the result of a mixture of inflammation and fibrosis: knowing the prevalent nature could be a turning point for CD management. Subjects with strictures with predominant inflammation can potentially be managed with medical therapy, whereas patients with prevalent fibrosis frequently need endoscopic dilatation or surgery, in particular in the presence of obstructive symptoms [13].

In this setting, stenosis characterization with the description of bowel wall signals could be helpful. In a study directed by Maconi et al. [14] the loss of stratification in the bowel with hypoechoic pattern wall was associated to inflammatory stenosis, while a stratified pattern, with an increase in submucosal echogenicity, was typical of fibrotic component, as evident defined by resection specimens (Figs. 4.8 and 4.9). This could be due to the deposition of collagen in the submucosal layer. The same authors assessed the differences in sensitivity of stenosis detection on the basis of location: it was 84.6% for ileal ones and 58.8% for colonic ones [15].

Moreover, several studies have revealed that the degree of vascularization on colour Doppler and *contrast-enhanced ultrasonography* (*CEUS*)

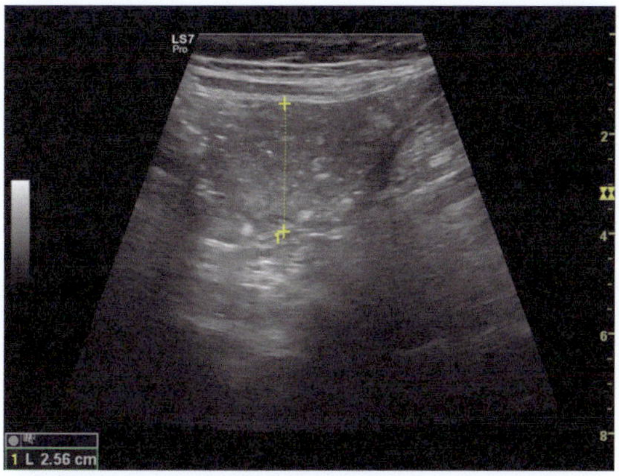

Fig. 4.4 Details of proximal dilatation

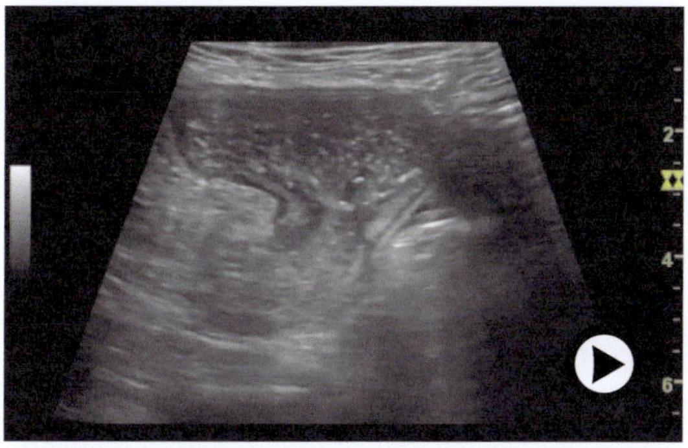

Fig. 4.5 Proximal dilatation (>25–30 mm) of the bowel is another parameter to identify a stenosis (▶ https://doi.org/10.1007/000-j21)

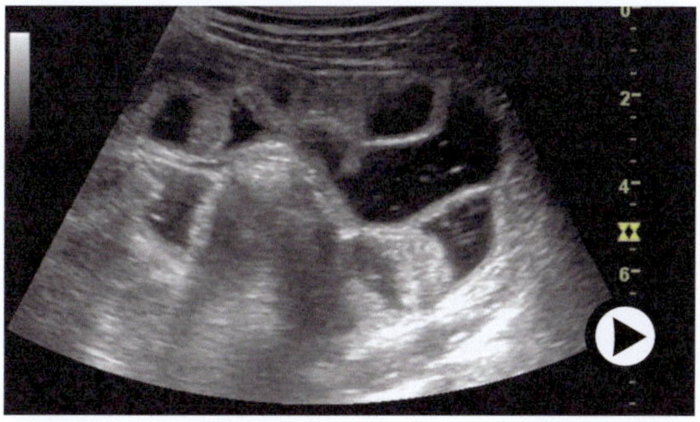

Fig. 4.6 Hyperperistalsis of the pre-stenotic gut (▶ https://doi.org/10.1007/000-j22)

is correlated with the histological degree of inflammation [16, 17] and could be useful to differentiate inflammatory from fibrostenotic lesions in CD. Most studies showed that the contrast enhancement of the bowel wall of inflamma-

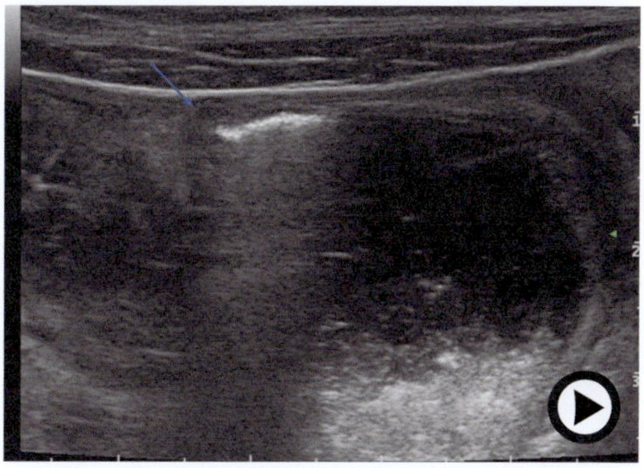

Fig. 4.7 Hydro-aerial levels detected in a dilated bowel loop proximal to a stenosis. Air is identified by the horizontal reverberation artifact and is positioned superiorly (arrow) (▶ https://doi.org/10.1007/000-j23)

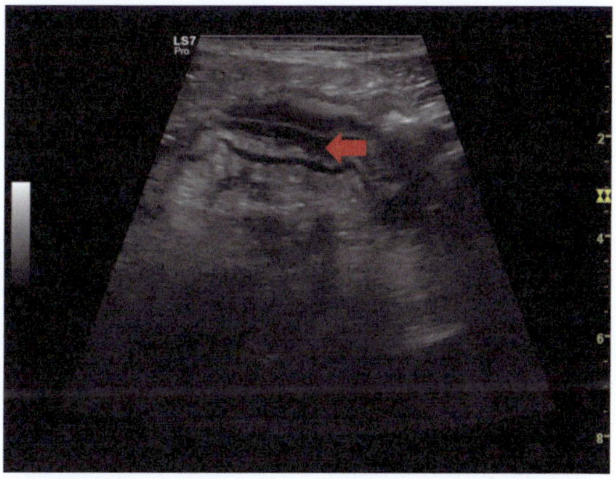

Fig. 4.8 Longitudinal image showing preserved bowel wall stratification with an increase in submucosal echogenicity (arrow), typical of fibrotic component

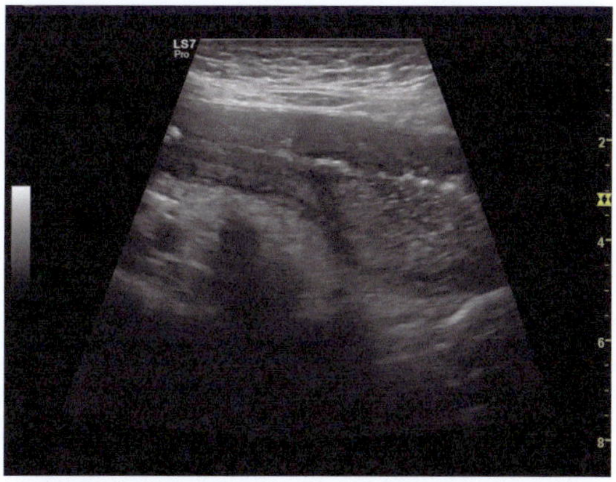

Fig. 4.9 Stenosis with loss of stratification (prevalent inflammatory stenosis)

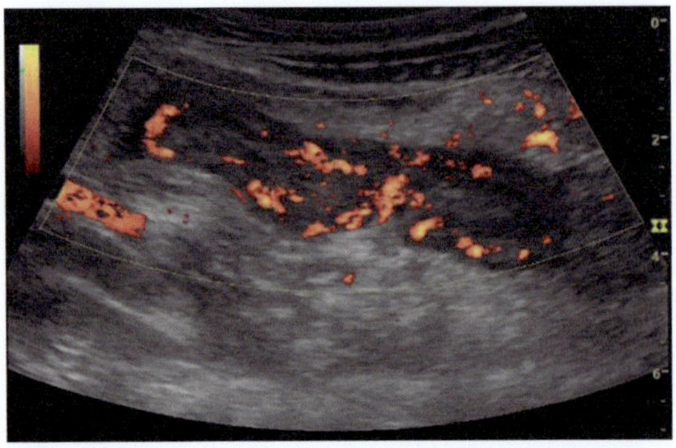

Fig. 4.10 Stenosis with vascular signals

tory stenosis (using surgical pathological specimens as the reference standard) is significantly superior compared to that of fibrotic strictures [18–21] (Fig. 4.10).

Some studies reported a significant correlation between the assessment of transabdominal bowel wall stiffness evaluated by *sonoelastography* and the amount of bowel fibrosis at histology [16–21]. This procedure evaluates the elastic properties of soft tissues by mechanical or acoustic stimulation: the tissue response is converted as an image with a scale of colours or as a quantitative measurement corresponding to the estimated stiffness value. The principal types of *sonoelastography* are strain elastography (SE) and shear wave elastography (SWE). Point-SWE (pSWE) assesses a quantitative value of a specific point of the studied tissue, while SWE reproduces a colour map that reflects the stiffness of a larger slice of the examined tissue. This technique has already been used in the diagnostic algorithms of diseases of the breast, liver, thyroid and pancreas, especially for neoplastic lesions [22]. In CD stenoses, higher SWE values have been reported in severe compared to mild and moderate fibrosis [20]. Data from a recent systematic review show that sonoelastography has an overall moderate-to-good accuracy in detecting fibrosis in CD patients, compared to histological specimens; moreover SWE perform better than other elastographic procedures [23].

The main limitations of *sonoelastography* and *CEUS* in this field are the high heterogeneity in results, the small sample size of the studies, the different methodologies in measurement, the absence of a validated scoring system and only a few use histopathology as the reference standard.

The combination of *CEUS* and sonoelastography may improve their accuracy in the characterization of CD-related stenosis [17, 24], but further studies are needed to confirm these evidences.

4.2 Fistulas

Patients with Crohn's disease (CD) can develop penetrating complications, including fistulas, which are more frequent in patients with ileal involvement [1]. Intestinal ultrasound (IUS) represents a valuable non-invasive technique for the identification and characterization of these complications. Deep ulcerations of the intestinal wall may give rise to extramural fissures, which are visualized as small hypoechoic irregularities of the bowel surface, in correspondence with hypoechoic segments of the bowel wall (Fig. 4.11). These fissures may evolve into sinus tracts and fistulas. Sinus tracts appear as linear hypoechoic extensions of inflammation, typically with a blind end or terminating within an inflammatory mesenteric mass (Fig. 4.12) [4, 5]. Abdominal fistulas are visualized as hypoechoic peri-intestinal segments or tracts and can be classified as internal or external. Internal fistulas may connect two bowel loops (entero-enteric) (Fig. 4.13 a, b), the bowel and the mesentery (entero-mesenteric), the abdominal wall (Fig. 4.14, Video 4.5), or adjacent abdominal organs such as the bladder (Fig. 4.15, Video 4.6) or the appendix (Fig. 4.16, Video 4.7). The presence of internal gaseous artifacts within these tracts may further support the diagnosis of fistulizing disease.

They are also classified as simple or complex. Simple fistulas are a single tract that connects bowel to another organ or abdominal surface; complex ones are multiple tracts that involve different structures and may show a star or asterisk configuration.

The US diagnostic criteria of sinus tracts and fistulas are: hypoechoic lines or tracts between ileal loops with or without internal hyperecho-

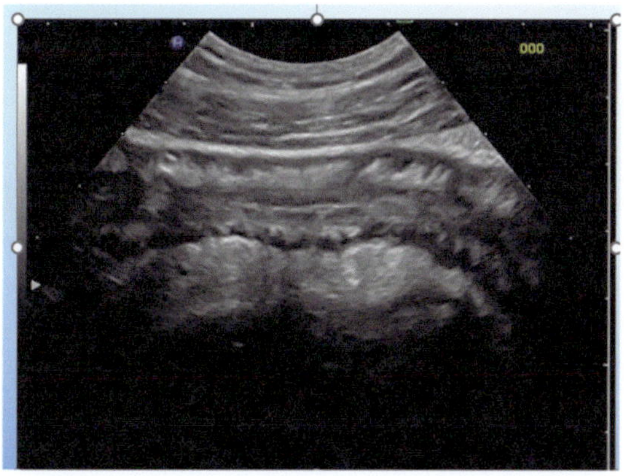

Fig. 4.11 An irregular profile of the ileal loop is visible, caused by multiple fissures

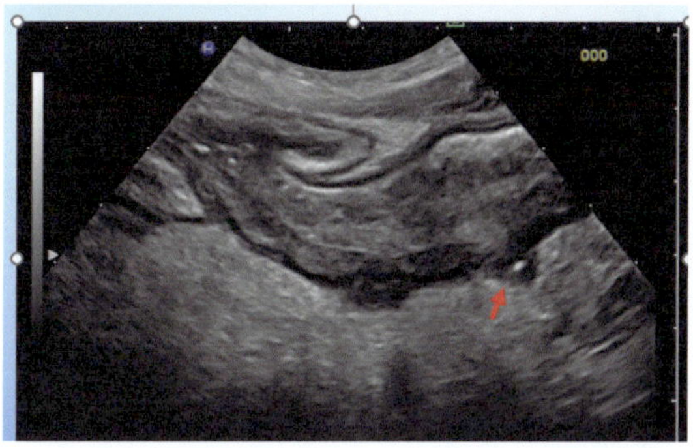

Fig. 4.12 Hypoechoic extensions of inflammation with a blind end and air inside, corresponding to a sinus tract (red arrow)

genic spots due to gaseous artifacts; hypoechoic tracts that originate from inflamed wall with or without gas within; hypoechoic peri-intestinal areas with a diameter <2 cm [4].

According to Pruijt et al., IUS's pooled sensitivity and specificity are 67 and 97%, even if not all the papers evaluated surgery as a reference standard [6].

The ingestion of polyethylene glycol (PEG) solution (500–800 mL) drunk approximately 30 min before IUS (small intestine contrast US; SICUS) has been shown to improve the sensitivity of IUS in the detection of fistulas, maybe because of a good definition of extraluminal complications consequent to PEG intake [8–10]. SICUS's pooled sensitivity and specificity in the diagnosis of fistulas are 90 and 94% [6].

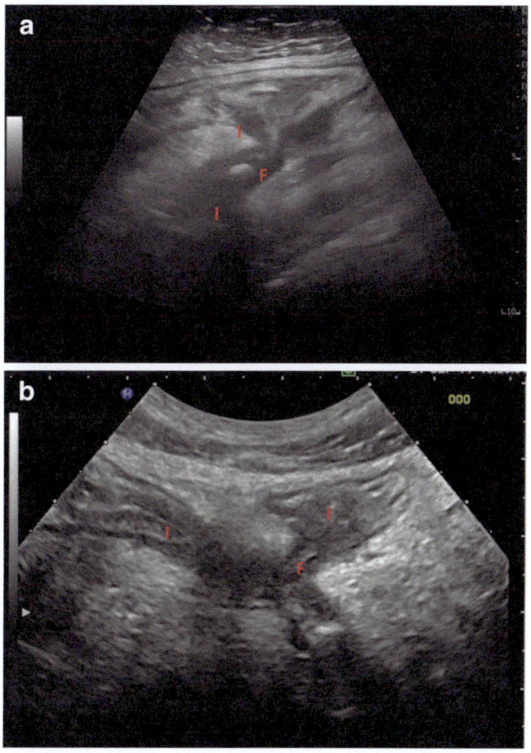

Fig. 4.13 Hypoechoic fistulous tract (F) connecting two ileal loops (I)

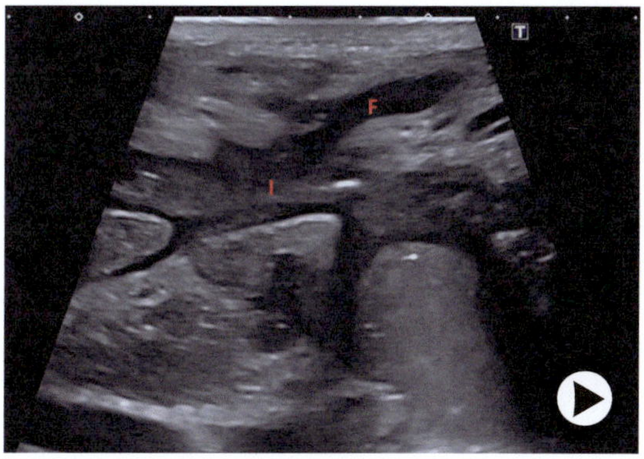

Fig. 4.14 Hypoechoic fistulous (F) tract extending from the intestinal loop (I) to the cutaneous surface (▶ https://doi.org/10.1007/000-j24)

Some studies have estimated the concordance of IUS with other radiologic techniques, such as computed tomography enteroclysis and magnetic resonance enterography (MRE) [12, 25]. IUS showed fair concordance with MRI in fistulas

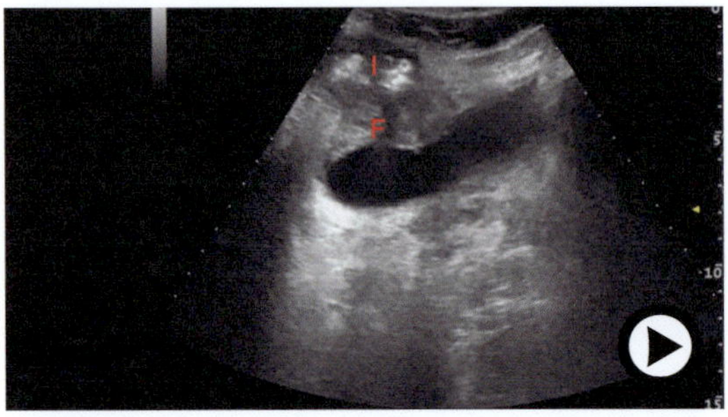

Fig. 4.15 Hypoechoic fistulous (F) tract extending from the intestinal loop (I) to the bladder (▶ https://doi.org/10.1007/000-j20)

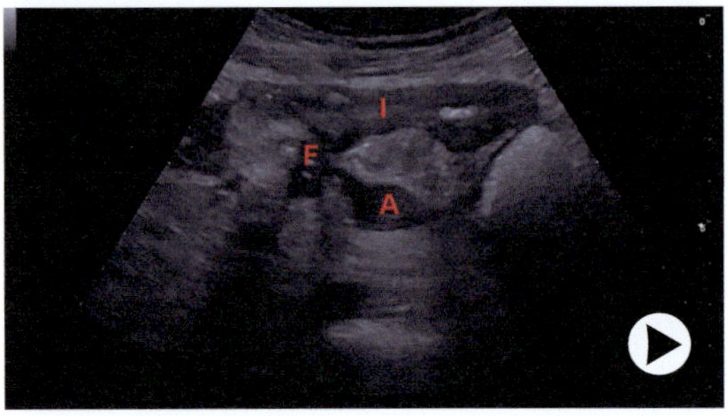

Fig. 4.16 Hypoechoic fistulous (F) tract extending from the intestinal loop (I) to the appendix (A) (▶ https://doi.org/10.1007/000-j26)

recognition ($k = 0.67$, $p = 0.01$) [12]; in a recent work IUS presented high sensitivity and specificity with 98% diagnostic accuracy compared to MRI in fistulas detection [25].

Moreover, fistulas are histologically characterized by degree of vascularization, which may explain their visualization by power Doppler US, as presented in a study by Maconi et al. [26]. Even in another work [27] power Doppler and CEUS are used to strengthen the diagnostic accuracy of IUS and to detect early and small inflammatory lesions (mean size of 18.5 mm), before developing into a fistula.

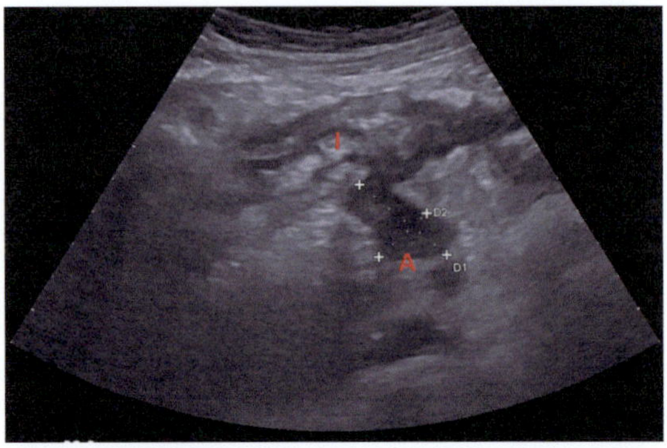

Fig. 4.17 Abscess (A) appears as an irregularly margined hypoechoic area in communication with a bowel loop (I)

4.3 Abscesses

Abscesses are other extramural complications of CD, evident in up to 30% of subjects with CD [1].

The US diagnostic criteria of abscesses are: hypo-anechoic lesions containing gaseous/liquid artifacts, regular or irregular wall, posterior enhancement, absence of peripheral/internal colour Doppler signals [4] (Figs. 4.17 and 4.18a, b).

IUS's pooled sensitivity and specificity in the detection of abscesses are 87 and 95% [6].

Abscesses and inflammatory masses may appear similar on IUS. CEUS and Doppler are helpful techniques in the distinction of these two kind of lesions [19, 28]. In fact they can show diffusely increased vascularization in inflammatory mass (Fig. 4.19, Video 4.8; Fig. 4.20, Video 4.9), while in case of an abscess it is visible only in the peripheral zone and not in the central one due to the presence of fluid collection (Fig. 4.21, Video 4.10; Fig. 4.22, Video 4.11).

A limit of standard IUS is the difficult detection of deep pelvic or intra- and retroperitoneal abscesses. This can be due to overlying bowel gas that may hide structures located between intestinal

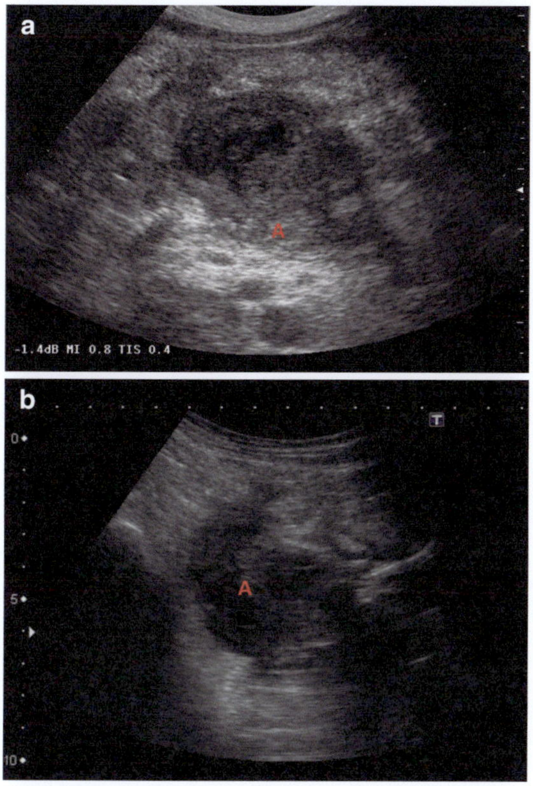

Fig. 4.18 Abscess (A) appears as a heterogeneous hypoechoic area with ill-defined margins

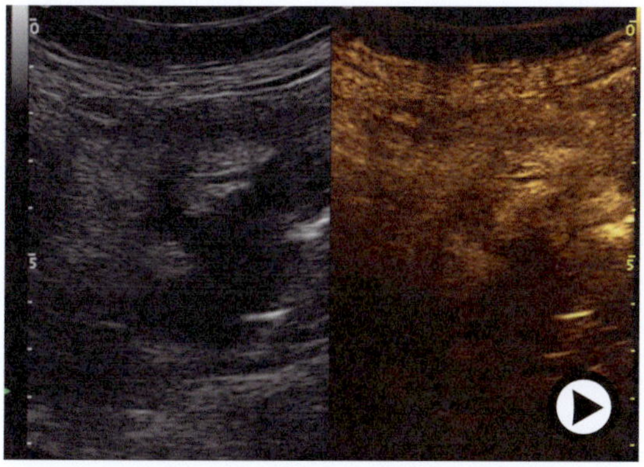

Fig. 4.19 Contrast-enhanced imaging reveals a hypo-anechoic formation on the left, exhibiting a mildly hypovascular pattern in the central region, without avascular areas suggestive of abscesses (▶ https://doi.org/10.1007/000-j27)

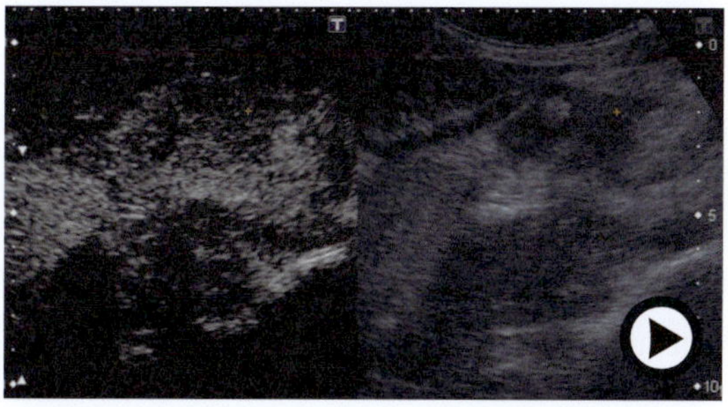

Fig. 4.20 Contrast-enhanced study shows the perianastomotic hypoechoic formation on the right (caliper) exhibiting a heterogeneous hypovascular pattern, with no avascular areas suggestive of abscesses (▶ https://doi.org/10.1007/000-j28)

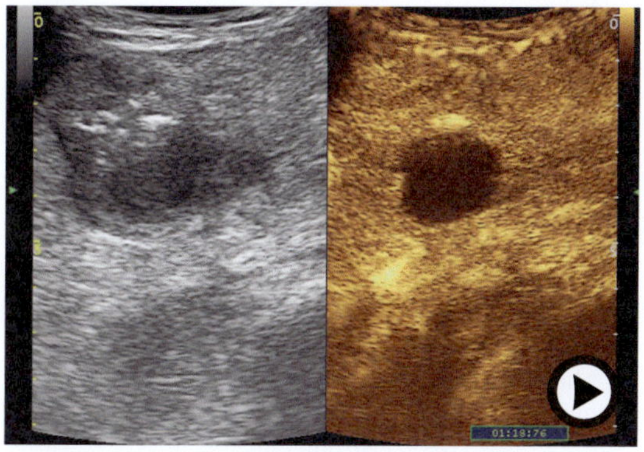

Fig. 4.21 Contrast-enhanced study reveals a hypoechoic formation on the left, displaying a completely avascular central area on CEUS, characteristic of an abscess collection (▶ https://doi.org/10.1007/000-j29)

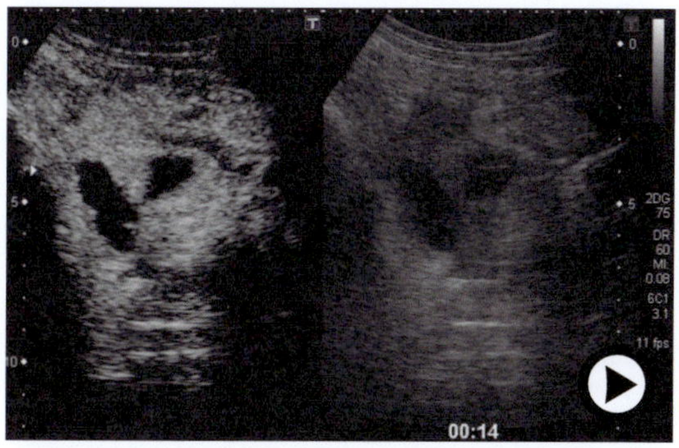

Fig. 4.22 Contrast-enhanced study shows the hypoechoic formation on the right, revealing two central completely avascular areas on CEUS, consistent with abscesses (▶ https://doi.org/10.1007/000-j2a)

loops or lying deep in the pelvis [8]. In this setting, Pallotta et al. showed increased sensitivity for SICUS in the detection of intra-abdominal masses; the distension of intestinal lumen after oral contrast may result in better differentiation between a bowel loop and an abscess [14]. SICUS's pooled sensitivity and specificity in the detection of these lesions are 91 and 97% [6].

Even in the diagnosis of abscesses many studies that evaluated the performance of different images techniques, IUS showed very good concordance with CT/MRI in the detection of these masses, as we can find in different works [8, 12].

References

1. Cosnes J, Gower-Rousseau C, Seksik P, et al. Epidemiology and natural history of inflammatory bowel diseases. Gastroenterology. 2011;140:1785–94.
2. Cosnes J, Cattan S, Blain A, et al. Long-term evolution of disease behaviour of Crohn's disease. Inflamm Bowel Dis. 2002;8:244–50.
3. Ismail MS, Charabaty A. Management of Crohn's stricture: medical, endoscopic and surgical therapies. Frontline Gastroenterol. 2022;13(6):524–30.
4. Maconi G, Nylund K, Ripolles T, et al. EFSUMB recommendations and clinical guidelines for intestinal ultrasound (GIUS) in inflammatory bowel diseases. Ultraschall Med. 2018;39(3):304–17.
5. Kucharzik T, Tielbeek J, Carter D, et al. ECCO-ESGAR topical review on optimizing reporting for cross-sectional imaging in inflammatory bowel disease. J Crohns Colitis. 2022;16(4):523–43.
6. Pruijt MJ, de Voogd FAE, Montazeri NSM, et al. Diagnostic accuracy of intestinal ultrasound in the detection of intra-abdominal complications in Crohn's disease: a systematic review and meta-analysis. J Crohns Colitis. 2024;18(6):958–72.
7. Parente F, Greco S, Molteni M, et al. Oral contrast enhanced bowel ultrasonography in the assessment of small intestine Crohn's disease. A prospective comparison with conventional ultrasound, × ray studies, and ileocolonoscopy. Gut. 2004;53:1652–7.
8. Pallotta N, Vincoli G, Montesani C, et al. Small intestine contrast ultrasonography (SICUS) for the detection of small bowel complications in Crohn's disease: a prospective comparative study versus intraoperative findings. Inflamm Bowel Dis. 2012;18(1):74–84.
9. Calabrese E, Zorzi F, Onali S, et al. Accuracy of small-intestine contrast ultrasonography, compared with computed tomography enteroclysis, in characterizing lesions in patients with Crohn's disease. Clin Gastroenterol Hepatol. 2013;11:950–5.
10. Kumar S, Hakim A, Alexakis C, et al. Small intestinal contrast ultrasonography for the detection of small bowel complications in Crohn's disease: correlation with intraoperative findings and magnetic resonance enterography: small intestinal contrast ultrasonography in Crohn's disease. J Gastroenterol Hepatol. 2015;30(1):86–91.
11. Onali S, Calabrese E, Petruzziello C, et al. Small intestine contrast ultrasonography vs computed tomography enteroclysis for assessing ileal Crohn's disease. WJG. 2012;18(42):6088.
12. Castiglione F, Mainenti PP, De Palma GD, et al. Noninvasive diagnosis of small bowel Crohn's disease: direct comparison of bowel sonography and magnetic resonance enterography. Inflamm Bowel Dis. 2013;19(5):991–8.
13. Adamina M, Bonovas S, Raine T, et al. ECCO guidelines on therapeutics in Crohn's disease: surgical treatment. J Crohns Colitis. 2020;14(2):155–68.
14. Maconi G, Carsana L, Fociani P, et al. Small bowel stenosis in Crohn's disease: clinical, biochemical and ultrasonographic evaluation of histological features. Alim Pharmacol Ther. 2003;18:749–56.
15. Maconi G, Bollani S, Bianchi PG. Ultrasonographic detection of intestinal complications in Crohn's disease. Dig Dis Sci. 1996;41:1643–8.
16. Fraquelli M, Branchi F, Cribiù FM, et al. The role of ultrasound elasticity imaging in predicting ileal fibrosis in Crohn's disease patients. Inflamm Bowel Dis. 2015;21:2605–12.
17. Lu C, Gui X, Chen W, et al. Ultrasound shear wave and contrast enhancement: effective biomarkers in Crohn's disease strictures. Inflamm Bowel Dis. 2017;23:421–30.
18. Baumgart DC, Müller HP, Grittner U, et al. US-based Real-time elastography for the detection of fibrotic gut tissue in patients with stricturing Crohn disease. Radiology. 2015;275:889–99.
19. Serra C, Rizzello F, Pratico C, et al. Real-time elastography for the detection of fibrotic and inflammatory tissue in patients with stricturing Crohn's disease. J Ultrasound. 2017;20:273–84.
20. Chen YJ, Mao R, Li XH, et al. Real-time shear wave ultrasound elastography differentiates fibrotic from inflammatory strictures in patients with Crohn's disease. Inflamm Bowel Dis. 2018;24:2183–90.
21. Ding SS, Fang Y, Wan J, et al. Usefulness of strain elastography, ARFI imaging, and point shear wave elastography for the assessment of Crohn disease strictures. J Ultrasound Med. 2019;38:2861–70.
22. Cosgrove D, Barr R, Bojunga J, et al. WFUMB guidelines and recommendations on the clinical use of ultrasound elastography: Part 4 Thyroid. Ultrasound Med Biol. 2017;43:4–26.

23. Dal Buono A, Faita F, Peyrin-Biroulet L, et al. Ultrasound elastography in inflammatory bowel diseases: a systematic review of accuracy compared with histopathological assessment. J Crohns Colitis. 2022;16(10):1637–46.
24. Quaia E, Gennari AG, van Beek EJR. Differentiation of inflammatory from fibrotic ileal strictures among patients with Crohn's disease through analysis of time-intensity curves obtained after microbubble contrast agent injection. Ultrasound Med Biol. 2017;43:1171–8.
25. Allocca M, Fiorino G, Bonifacio C, et al. Comparative accuracy of bowel ultrasound versus magnetic resonance enterography in combination with colonoscopy in assessing Crohn's disease and guiding clinical decision making. J Crohns Colitis. 2018;12(11):1280–7.
26. Maconi G, Sampietro GM, Russo A, et al. The vascularity of internal fistulas in Crohn's disease: an in vivo power Doppler ultrasonography assessment. Gut. 2002;50:496–500.
27. Esteban JM, Aleixandre A, Hurtado MJ, Maldonado L, Mora FJ, Nogues E. Contrast-enhanced power Doppler ultrasound in the diagnosis and follow-up of inflammatory abdominal masses in Crohn's disease. Eur J Gastroenterol Hepatol. 2003;15:253–9.
28. Ripolles T, Rausell N, Paredes JM, et al. Effectiveness of contrast-enhanced ultrasound for characterisation of intestinal inflammation in Crohn's disease: a comparison with surgical histopathology analysis. J Crohns Colitis. 2013;7(120–8):38.

5 Ultrasound Evaluation in Ulcerative Colitis: Role of Bowel Ultrasound in Identifying Ulcerative Colitis

Fabrizio Bossa, Francesco Cocomazzi, and Lorenzo Maria Vetrone

5.1 Introduction

Ulcerative colitis (UC) is a chronic inflammatory bowel disease (IBD) of unknown etiology that results in inflammatory involvement of the large intestine [1]. UC mainly affects the more superficial layers of the intestinal wall (mucosa and submucosa) and is characterized by continuous involvement of the large intestine starting from the rectum and extending proximally till the cecum, and sometimes to the terminal ileum (so-called backwash ileitis).

Supplementary Information The online version contains supplementary material available at https://doi.org/10.1007/978-3-032-11418-1_5. The videos can be accessed individually by clicking the DOI link in the accompanying figure caption or by scanning this link with the SN More Media App.

F. Bossa (✉) · F. Cocomazzi · L. M. Vetrone
Division of Gastroenterology and Digestive Endoscopy, Fondazione IRCCS "Casa Sollievo della Sofferenza", San Giovanni Rotondo, Italy
e-mail: f.bossa@operapadrepio.it

5.2 Role of Ultrasonography in Ulcerative Colitis Diagnosis and Follow-Up

Typical symptoms of UC include diarrhea, rectal tenesmus, and hematochezia. The diagnosis of UC is based on a combination of clinical, laboratory, radiological, endoscopic, and histological investigations [2]. The presence of blood in the stool makes endoscopic examination with multiple biopsies mandated.

The severity of inflammation is usually classified into three stages: mild, moderate, and severe using different endoscopic scores, among which the most popular is the endoscopic Mayo score [3]. In Fig. 5.1, we showed the endoscopic Mayo score with corresponding endoscopic images.

The intestinal (bowel) ultrasound (IUS) can accurately study the colon and identify signs of inflammation, and it is useful in case of suspected UC (for example, in cases of chronic diarrhea without blood in the stool). In addition, bowel ultrasonography allows assessing the extent of the inflammation non-invasively.

In the follow-up of UC patients, IUS allows assessment of disease activity, and it is a helpful

F. Terracciano et al. (eds.), *Bowel Ultrasound Compared with Endoscopy*,
https://doi.org/10.1007/978-3-032-11418-1_5

Score	Disease activity	Endoscopic features
0	Normal orinactive	None
1	Mild	Erythema, decreased vascular pattern, mild friability
2	Moderate	Marked erythema, absence of vascular pattern, friability, erosions
3	Severe	Spontaneous bleeding, ulcerations

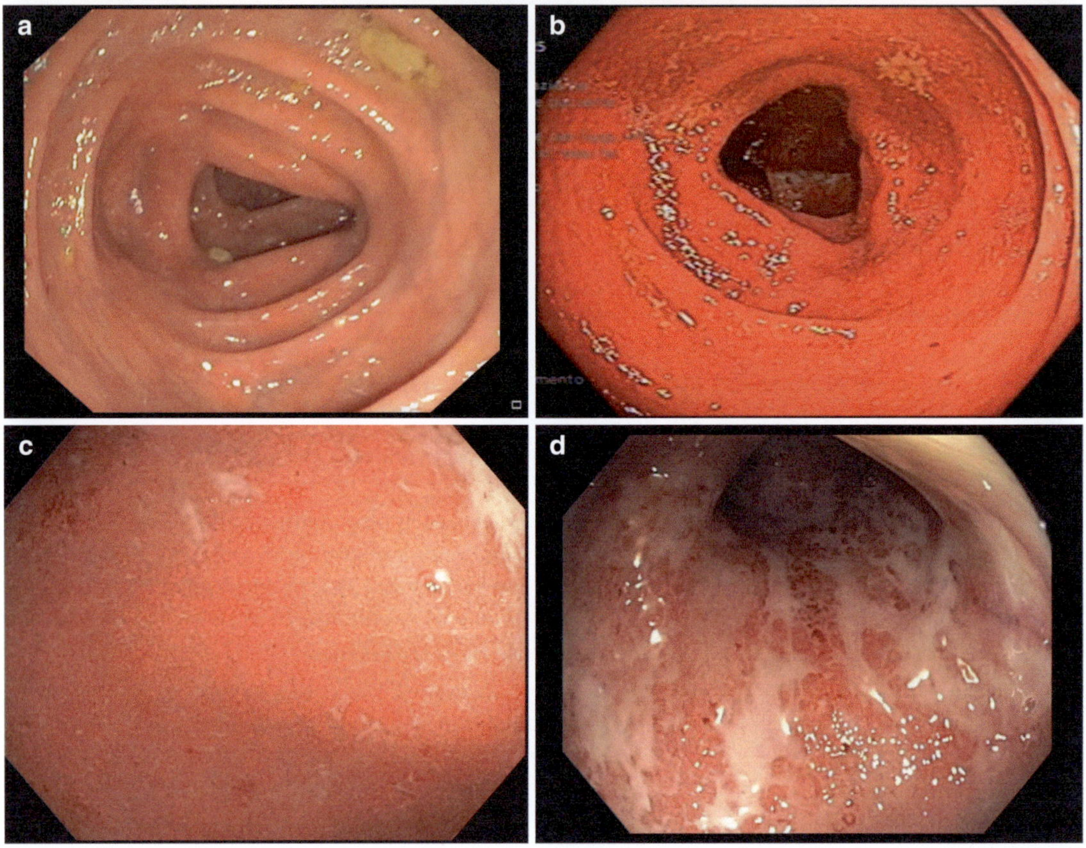

Fig. 5.1 Mayo endoscopic score for ulcerative colitis (UC). (**a**) UC in remission (Mayo 0); (**b**) UC with mild activity (Mayo 1); (**c**) UC with moderate activity (Mayo 2); (**d**) UC with severe activity (Mayo 3)

non-invasive tool for evaluating the response to the therapy [4]. In addition, IUS allows the detection of some complications such as colonic stenosis, colorectal cancer, or toxic megacolon.

5.3 Ultrasonographic Features of UC

The main ultrasound characteristics of UC are loss of colonic haustration, continuous colonic involvement, and increased wall thickness (≥4 mm). In Fig. 5.2, we depicted the main ultrasonographic features of UC. In contrast to Crohn's disease, the thickening of the wall affects

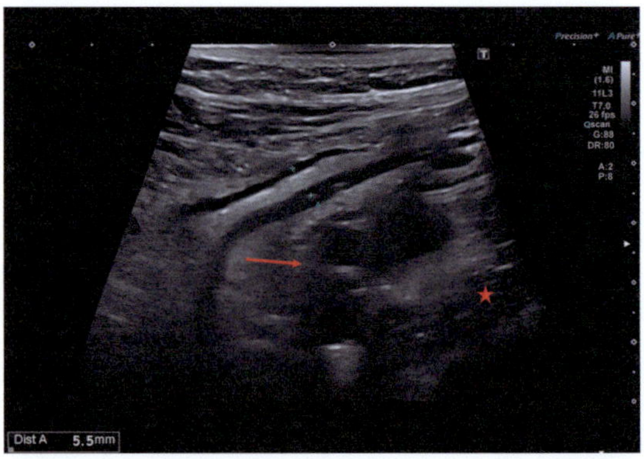

Fig. 5.2 Linear probe positioned in the left iliac fossa. Anatomical landmarks are identified: iliac vessels (red arrows) and the psoas muscle (asterisk). The sigmoid colon shows thickened walls (5.5 mm), with increased prominence of the hyperechoic submucosal layer and loss of normal haustration

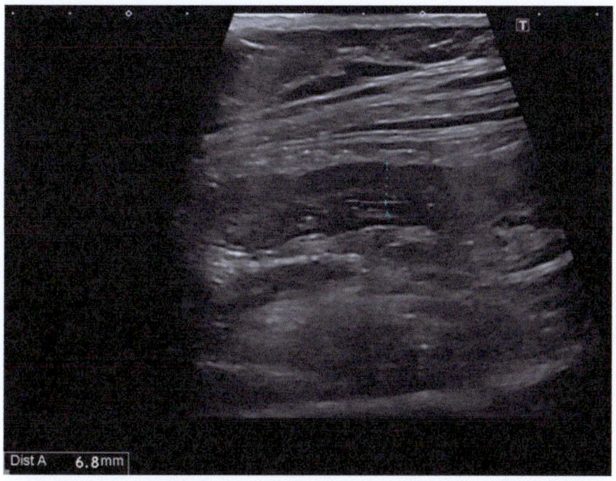

Fig. 5.3 Descending colon of patients with severe acute ulcerative colitis. Bowel thickened (7 mm) and loss of stratification (hypoechoic pattern)

the more superficial layers (mucosa and submucosa) and it is usually less than 5 mm. Rarely, the bowel wall may reach or exceed 7 mm. The stratification of the intestinal wall layers is usually preserved. However, in severe activity, wall thickening may involve all layers with a loss of parietal stratification, usually associated with a wall thickening of more than 7 mm (Fig. 5.3). Other ultrasound findings are enlarged mesenteric lymph nodes (short axis >5 mm), and mesenteric hypertrophy (defined as the presence of a hyperechoic area surrounding the pathologic intestinal wall), as showed in the Fig. 5.4.

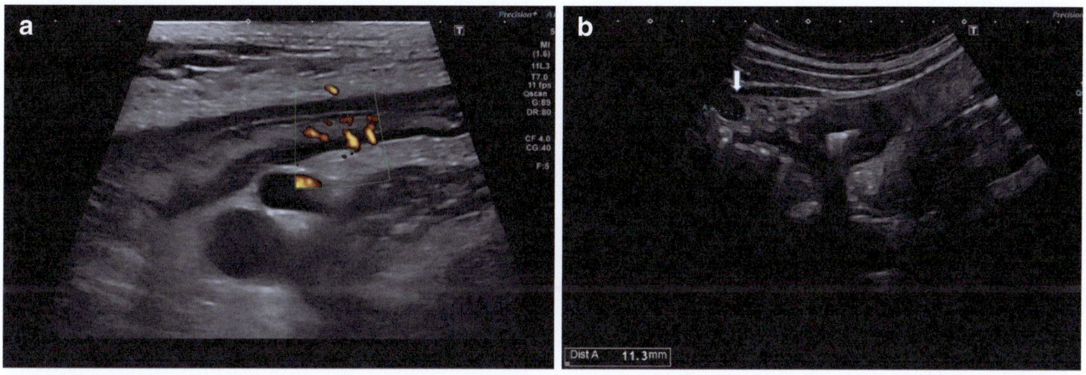

Fig. 5.4 Sigmoid colon of a patient with active UC. Mesenteric hypertrophy (**a**) appears as hyperechoic tissue surrounding the bowel loop. (**b**) Reactive lymph node (arrow) hypoechoic oval or rounded

5.4 Role of IUS in Assessing Disease Activity

The grade of activity influence management and treatment modality of UC patients. Despite colonoscopy being the reference examination to evaluate the activity of UC [5], IUS can accurately evaluate intestinal inflammation allowing esteem for the extension and the activity of UC except for the rectum [6–8]. However, transperineal ultrasound (TPUS) of the rectum allows to assess disease activity in this segment virtually in all patients, both adult and pediatric [9, 10].

TPUS is performed in the Sims position. The probe is placed on the perineal region allowing to study the anal canal, the anal sphincters, the perineal spaces, and to assess the walls of the distal rectum. The value considered normal for wall thickness of the rectum is 4 mm.

The most significantly associated feature with inflammation is the thickness of the intestinal wall. The intra- and extramural blood flow assessment by color Doppler represents another sign significantly associated with grade of inflammation. The semi-quantitative Limberg score [11] is the most widely used for color Doppler assessment.

This correlation is mainly based on key ultrasonographic parameters such as bowel wall thickness and the presence of color Doppler signal, both of which increase in parallel with the severity of inflammation. Through these parameters, ultrasound can effectively differentiate between clinical or endoscopic remission and active disease. Moreover in 2018, a prospective study involved 53 UC patients who underwent IUS and colonoscopy to assess the concordance of the two techniques [12] in evaluating the inflammation. At the multivariable analysis, colon wall thickening (CWT) and colon wall flow (CWF) were significantly associated with endoscopic activity. The authors built an ultrasonography-based score to assess disease activity. A score ≥6.2 resulted in an indicator of endoscopic activity (Mayo endoscopic subscore ≥2), with a specificity of 100%. The score was then validated in a subsequent study in a different cohort of UC patients [13].

Despite these strengths, IUS does have some limitations. It may not always clearly distinguish between the different grades of endoscopic activity—Mayo 1, 2, and 3—particularly when attempting to separate mild from moderate inflammation. Figure 5.5 compares the different degrees of endoscopic disease activity with the corresponding ultrasound images (Figs. 5.6, Video 5.1; Fig. 5.7, Video 5.2; Figs. 5.8, 5.9; Fig. 5.10, Video 5.3).

In conclusion, while IUS cannot fully replace colonoscopy when a detailed endoscopic assessment is required, especially in cases where precise grading is necessary, it remains a highly useful method for monitoring disease activity and estimating endoscopic severity in daily clinical practice.

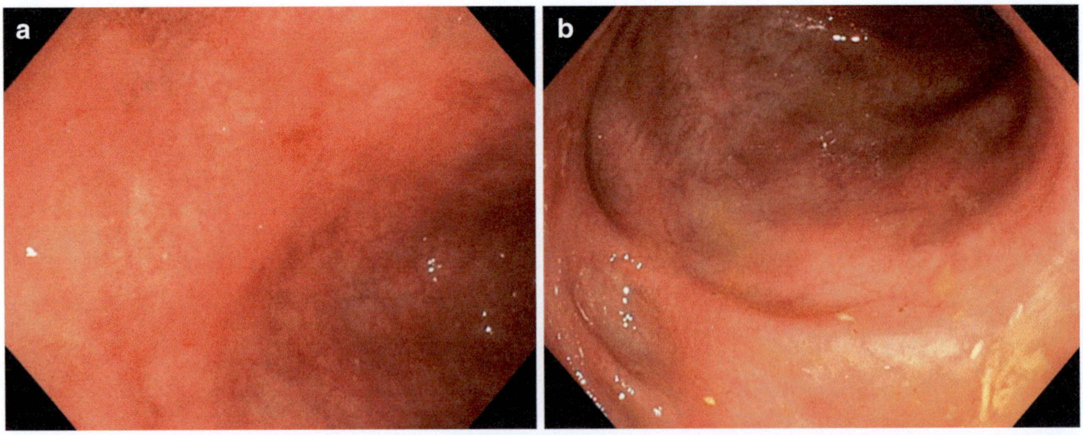

Fig. 5.5 Mild active ulcerative colitis (Mayo 1). Endoscopic images (**a** and **b**) show a colon with diffusely hyperemic and edematous mucosa, with no evidence of erosions and/or ulcers

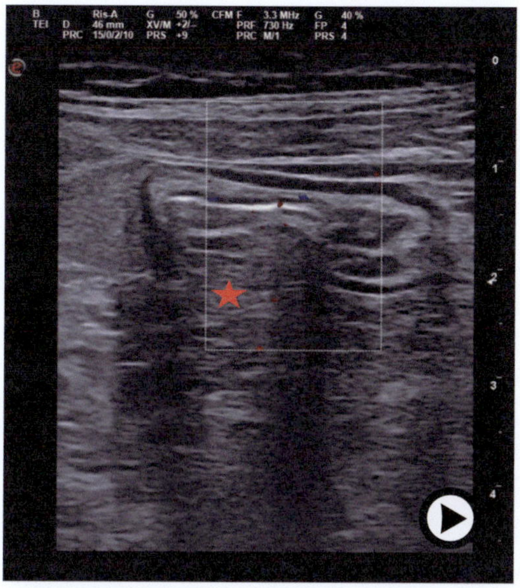

Fig. 5.6 Transverse section of the descending colon. The colonic wall is not thickened, and the luminal content is mixed, containing enteric material and air (horizontal reverberation artifact). A small reactive lymphadenopathy is present to the left of the bowel loop (▶ https://doi.org/10.1007/000-j2d)

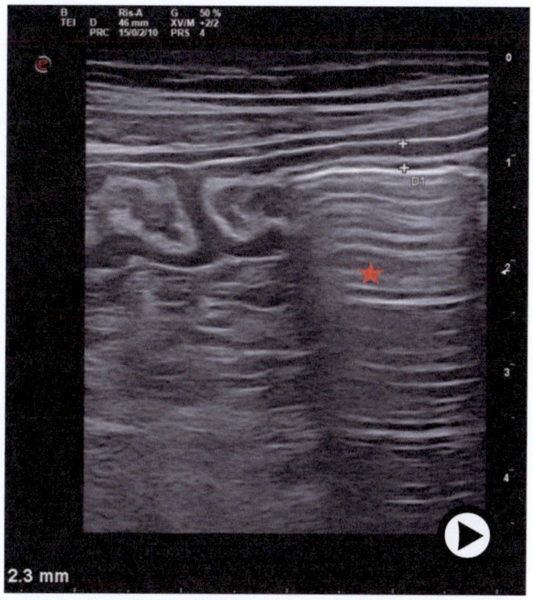

Fig. 5.7 Longitudinal section of the descending colon. The left colon shows a normal wall thickness, preserved wall stratification, increased of submucosa layer and less prominet haustration (▶ https://doi.org/10.1007/000-j2c)

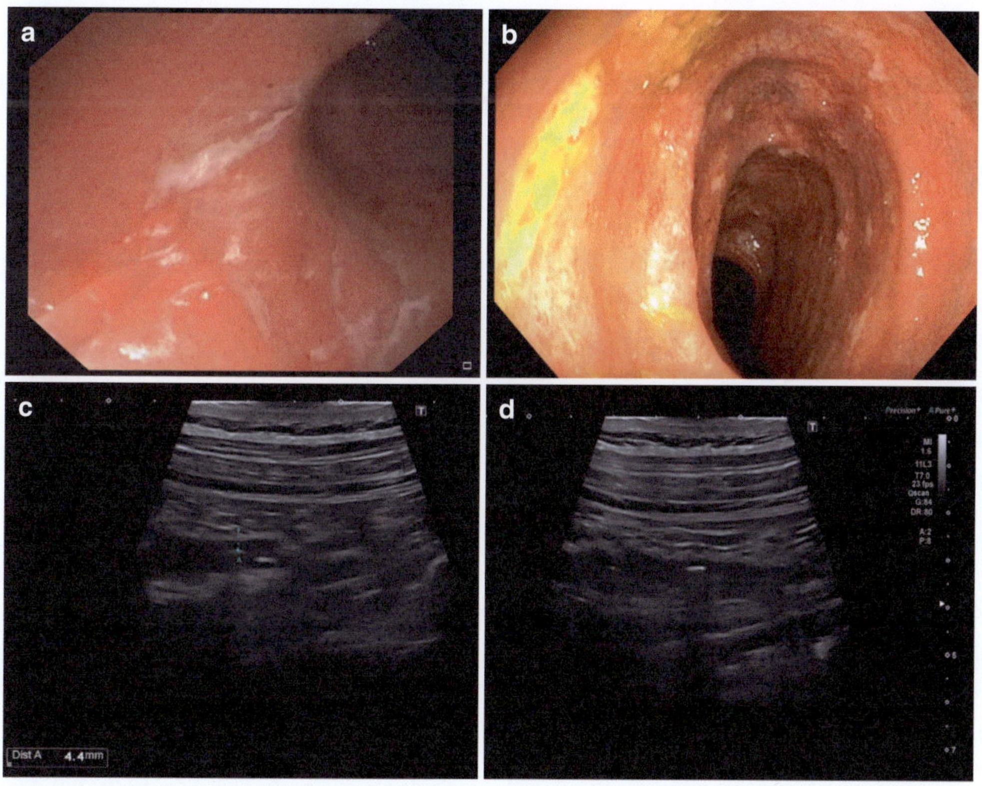

Fig. 5.8 Moderate active ulcerative colitis (Mayo 2). Mild erythema, edema, and minute mucosal erosions on colonoscopy (**a** and **b**). Corresponding ultrasound findings: bowel wall thickening (4.4 mm) with preserved stratification and loss of haustration (**c** and **d**)

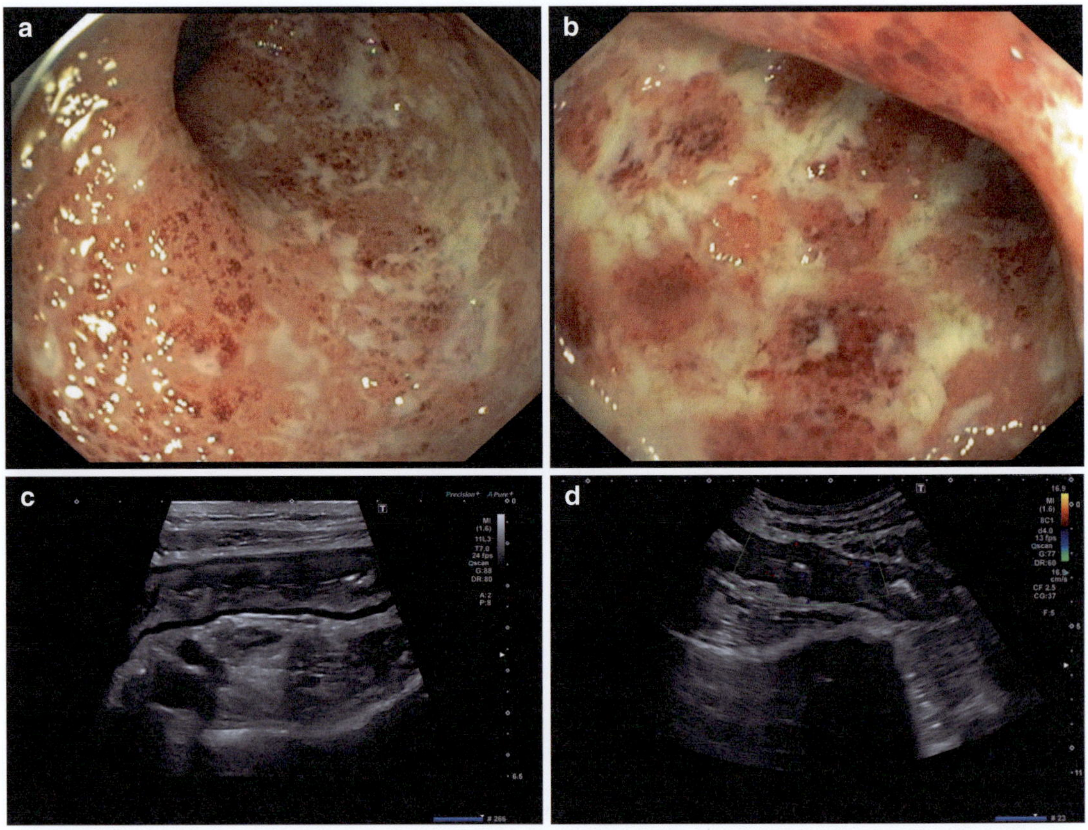

Fig. 5.9 Severe active ulcerative colitis (Mayo 3). In images **a** and **b**, the mucosa appears intensely and diffusely erythematous, friable with spontaneous bleeding, and shows multiple ulcerations and adherent mucus. The corresponding ultrasound findings include a parietal wall thickening of 8 mm with loss of stratification (**c**) and increased color Doppler signal (**d**)

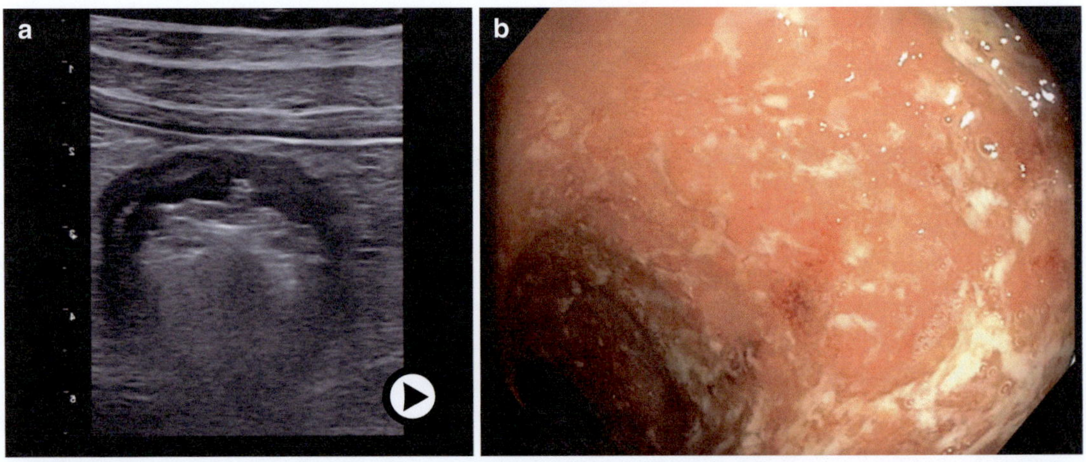

Fig. 5.10 Details in a patient with severe ulcerative colitis. (**a**) Presence of a hyperechoic intramural spot (arrow) suggestive of an intraparietal ulceration; the bowel wall appears thickened with loss of normal stratification, suggestive of severe active disease. (**b**) Corresponding endoscopic findings show diffusely erythematous mucosa with multiple ulcerations (▶ https://doi.org/10.1007/000-j2b)

5.5 Role of IUS in Assessing Response to Treatment

Good concordance between IUS and colonoscopy for the assessment of activity in UC is a prerequisite for the use of ultrasound for non-invasive assessment of response to therapy. A systematic review and expert consensus statement recently published, defined the IUS features for treatment response and remission in IBD [13]. Treatment response should be identified by reduction of bowel wall thickness (>2 mm or >1 mm when associated to one color Doppler signal reduction). The timing of evaluation is usually considered after 14 ± 2 weeks after the baseline evaluation. Transmural remission in ulcerative colitis is defined by bowel wall thickness ≤3 mm with normal color Doppler signal [14].

5.6 Role of IUS in the Differential Diagnosis with Other Colitis

Active UC cannot be distinguished from Crohn's disease by sonography unless the small bowel is involved. However, certain features can help in the differential diagnosis as in Crohn's disease wall thickening is usually more pronounced (>7 mm) [11]. In case of infectious enteritis, more mesenteric lymphonodes and fluid-filled small bowel loops with irregular peristalsis can be visualized [15]. Acute diverticulitis has a different clinical presentation from UC. The bowel ultrasound can show the thickening of the wall, usually with loss of normal stratification, mesenteric hypertrophy, and sometimes the presence of pericolic abscesses [16]. Ischemic colitis is characterized by segmental involvement of the colon, wall thickness, loss of wall layers differentiation, and typical absence of color Doppler signals [17]. Drug antibiotic-associated colitis usually presents as hypoechoic, pronounced thickening of the bowel wall [18]. Hypertrophy of the hypoechoic muscular layer of the bowel wall (so-called myochosis coli) associated with non-inflamed diverticula is a typical feature of chronic diverticular disease [19]. In all these cases, information from clinical history, radiological investigation, and laboratory tests are decisive for the correct diagnosis.

5.7 Role of IUS in the Complications of UC

Bowel perforation, intestinal hemorrhage, and toxic megacolon represent complications of severe acute UC. In addition, patients with long-standing disease have a higher risk of colorectal cancer than the general population. IUS has no role in cases of intestinal hemorrhage or perforation, whereas highly trained operators can recognize toxic megacolon. Megacolon should be suspected when there is a decrease in colonic wall thickness (<2 mm), associated with colonic dilatation (diameter >6 cm) and increased intraluminal fluid (Fig. 5.11, Video 5.4; Fig. 5.12) [20].

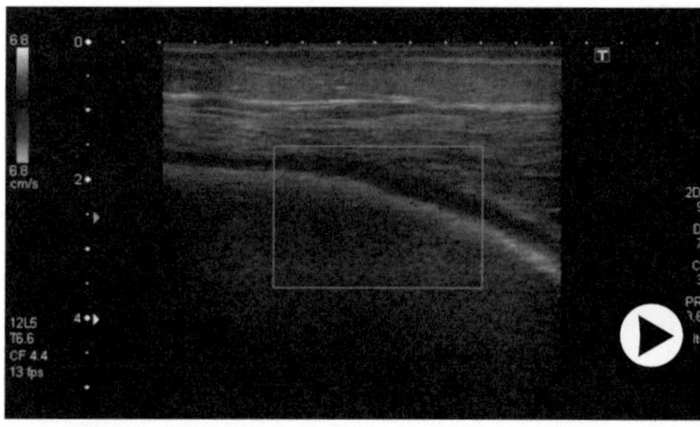

Fig. 5.11 The image shows a colon distended by significant gaseous content, with complete loss of haustration and a thin wall with absent vascular signals (▶ https://doi.org/10.1007/000-j2e)

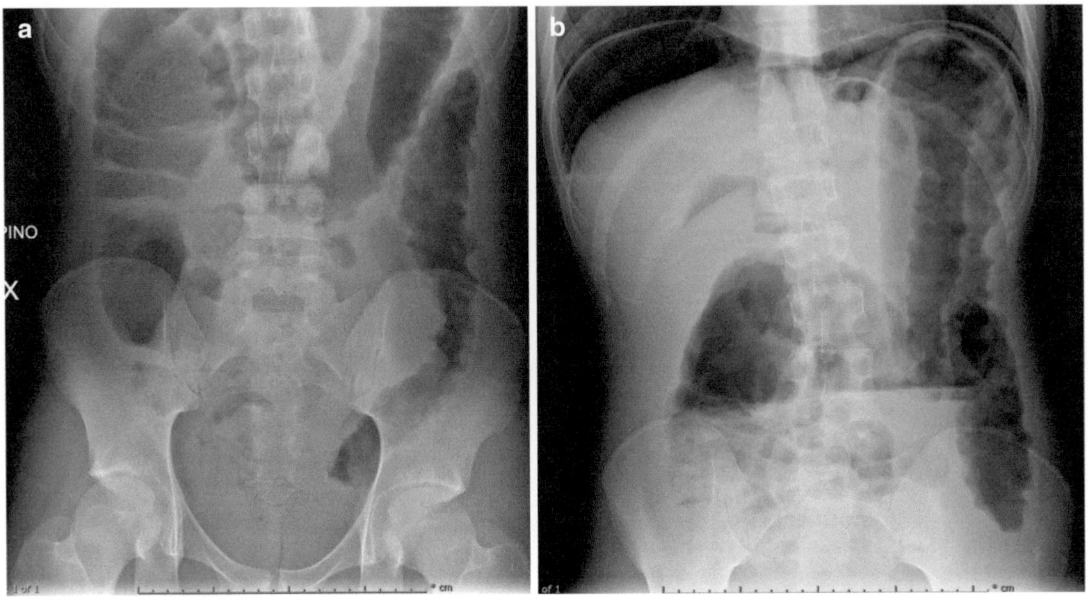

Fig. 5.12 (**a**) Abdominal X-ray showing marked colonic distension in the supine position. (**b**) Abdominal X-ray performed 3 days later showing free air in the abdomen

IUS can reveal irregular and eccentric thickenings of the intestinal wall with a pseudo-kidney appearance, which may be an expression of a neoplastic lesion.

References

1. Raine T, Bonovas S, Burisch J, et al. ECCO guidelines on therapeutics in ulcerative colitis: medical treatment. J Crohns Colitis. 2022;16(1):2–17.
2. Maaser C, Sturm A, Vavricka SR, et al. ECCO-ESGAR guideline for diagnostic assessment in IBD Part 1: Initial diagnosis, monitoring of known IBD, detection of complications. J Crohns Colitis. 2019;13:144–64K.
3. Schroeder KW, Tremaine WJ, Ilstrup DM. Coated oral 5-aminosalcylic acid therapy for mildly to moderately active ulcerative colitis. N Eng J Med. 1987;317(26):1625–9.
4. Johan FKF, Ilvemark A, Tawnya Hansen B, Goodsall TM, et al. Defining transabdominal intestinal ultrasound treatment response and remission in inflammatory bowel disease: systematic review and expert consensus statement. J Crohns Colitis. 2022:554–80.
5. Magro F, Gionchetti P, Eliakim R, et al. European Crohn's and Colitis Organisation [ECCO]. Third European evidence-based consensus on diagnosis and management of ulcerative colitis. Part 1: Definitions, diagnosis, extra-intestinal manifestations, pregnancy, cancer surveillance, surgery, and ileo-anal pouch disorders. J Crohns Colitis. 2017;11:649–70.
6. Maconi G, Ardizzone S, Parente F, Bianchi PG. Ultrasonography in the evaluation of extension, activity, and follow-up of ulcerative colitis. Scand J Gastroenterol. 1999;34:1103–7.
7. Antonelli E, Giuliano V, Casella G, et al. Ultrasonographic assessment of colonic wall in moderate-severe ulcerative colitis: comparison with endoscopic findings. Dig Liver Dis. 2011;43:703–6.
8. Parente F, Molteni M, Marino B, et al. Bowel ultrasound and mucosal healing in ulcerative colitis. Dig Dis. 2009;27:285–90.
9. Sagami S, Kobayashi T, Aihara K, et al. Transperineal ultrasound predicts endoscopic and histological healing in ulcerative colitis. Aliment Pharmacol Ther. 2020;51(12):1373–83.
10. Jimbo K, Hosoi K, Suzuki M, et al. Accuracy of transperineal ultrasonography for assessing rectal lesions in paediatric ulcerative colitis: a prospective study. J Crohns Colitis. 2024;17(7):1122–7.
11. Limberg B, Osswald B. Diagnosis and differential diagnosis of ulcerative colitis and Crohn's disease by hydrocolonic sonography. Am J Gastroenterol. 1994;89(7):1051–7.
12. Allocca M, Fiorino G, Bonovas S, et al. Accuracy of humanitas ultrasound criteria in assessing disease activity and severity in ulcerative colitis: a prospective study. J Crohns Colitis. 2018;12(12):1385–91.

13. Allocca M, Filippi E, Costantino A, et al. Milan ultrasound criteria are accurate in assessing disease activity in ulcerative colitis: external validation. United Eur Gastroenterol J. 2021;9(4):438–42.
14. Smith RL, Taylor KM, Friedman AB, et al. Early assessment with gastrointestinal ultrasound in patients hospitalised for a flare of ulcerative colitis and predicting the need for salvage therapy: a pilot study. Ultrasound Med Biol. 2021;47:1108–14.
15. Gutiérrez MÁM, Vigara AP, Nodal EM-O, et al. Value of abdominal ultrasound for evaluation of acute infectious ileitis in children. An Pediatr (Engl Ed). 2022;96(4):360–1.
16. Kwon LM, Lee K, Kim M-J, et al. Acute ileal diverticulitis: computed tomography and ultrasound findings. Diagnostics (Basel). 2023;13(8):1408.
17. Del Rosario M, Pastor-Juan TR, Martí-Bonmatí L, et al. Predictors of severity in ischemic colitis: usefulness of early ultrasonography. Eur J Radiol. 2017;96:21–6.
18. Wiener-Well Y, Kaloti S, Hadas-Halpern I. Ultrasound diagnosis of Clostridium difficile-associated diarrhea. Eur J Clin Microbiol Infect Dis. 2015;34(10):1975–8.
19. Berndt P, Niekisch G. Colonic diverticulitis. Primary clinical and ultrasound diagnosis – report of 47 cases from general practice. Z Arztl Fortbild Qualitatssich. 1997;91(2):171–4.
20. Maconi G, Sampietro GM, Ardizzone S, et al. Ultrasonographic detection of toxic megacolon in inflammatory bowel diseases. Dig Dis Sci. 2004;49:148–2.

6 Role of Intestinal Ultrasound in Assessing Disease Activity and in Evaluating the Response to Treatment in Ulcerative Colitis

Mariangela Allocca, Alessandra Zilli, and Federica Furfaro

6.1 Case 1

A 36-year-old woman with long-standing ulcerative pancolitis since 2007 associated with overlap syndrome (autoimmune hepatitis and primary sclerosing cholangitis), failure to infliximab, vedolizumab, and ustekinumab, on chronic steroid therapy for steroid dependence (Figs. 6.1, 6.2, 6.3 and 6.4, Video 6.1).

Supplementary Information The online version contains supplementary material available at https://doi.org/10.1007/978-3-032-11418-1_6. The videos can be accessed individually by clicking the DOI link in the accompanying figure caption or by scanning this link with the SN More Media App.

M. Allocca (✉)
Gastroenterology and Gastrointestinal Endoscopy Division, IRCCS San Raffaele Hospital, Milan, Italy

Faculty of Medicine and Surgery, Vita-Salute San Raffaele University, Milan, Italy

A. Zilli
Gastroenterology and Gastrointestinal Endoscopy Division, IRCCS San Raffaele Hospital, Milan, Italy

F. Furfaro
Gastroenterology and Gastrointestinal Endoscopy Division, IRCCS San Raffaele Hospital, Milan, Italy

Faculty of Medicine and Surgery, Vita-Salute San Raffaele University, Milan, Italy

Gastroenterology Unit, Istituti Ospedalieri Bergamaschi, Zingonia, Bergamo, Italy

F. Terracciano et al. (eds.), *Bowel Ultrasound Compared with Endoscopy*,
https://doi.org/10.1007/978-3-032-11418-1_6

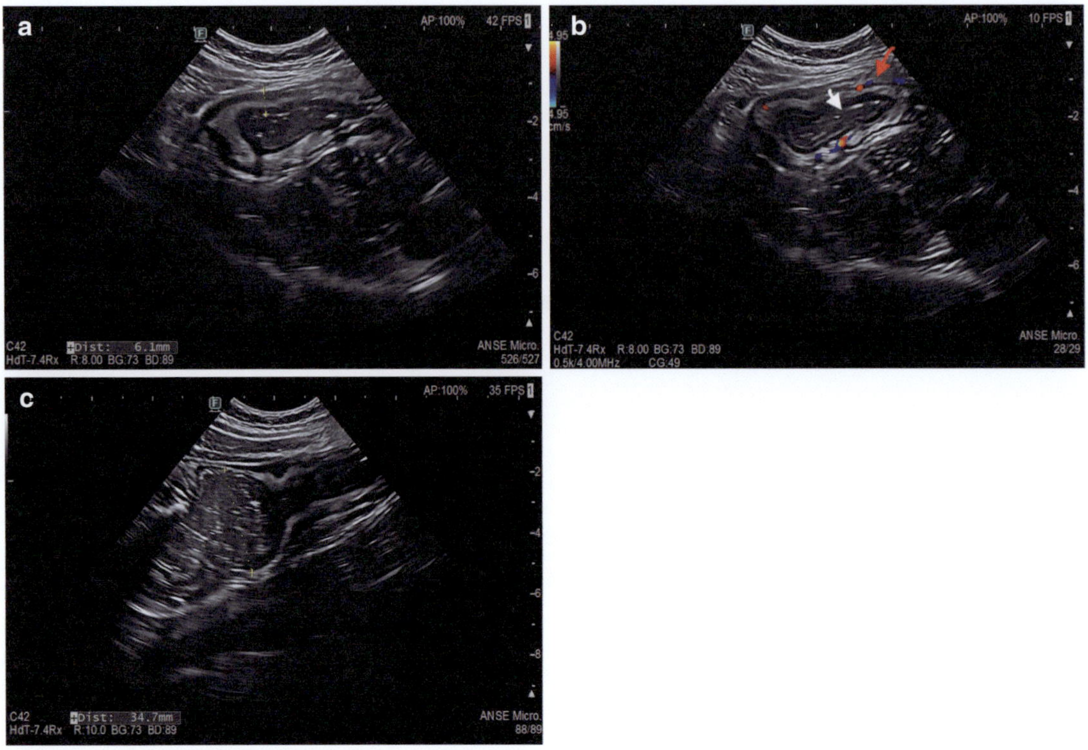

Fig. 6.1 Intestinal ultrasound. Thickening of bowel wall in the cecum (**a**) with normal stratification, echo pattern, increased vascularization at color Doppler (**b**) with vessels going outside the bowel wall (red arrow), irregular interface between the lumen and mucosal layers for presence of pseudo polyps and microulcerations (white arrow) and mild dilation with loss of haustration in the ascending colon (**c**), which is distended by feces

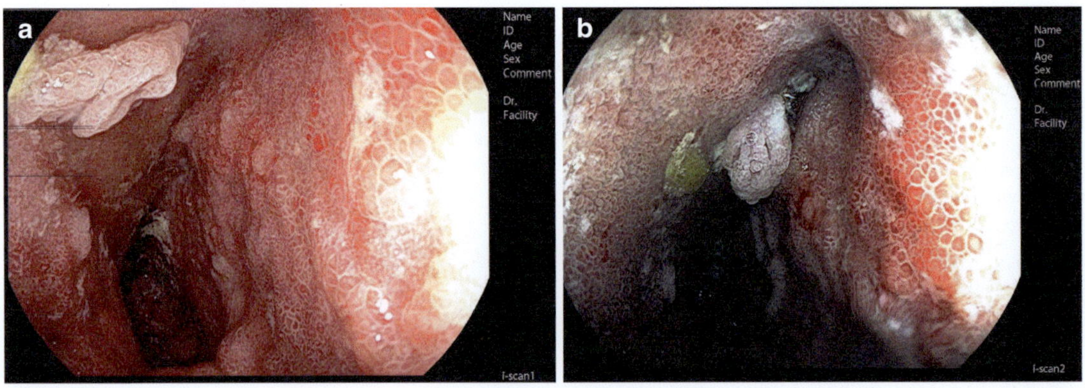

Fig. 6.2 Endoscopy. The right colon appears tubulized, markedly hyperemic, fragile, and easily bleeding, with scattered erosions and inflammatory sessile pseudo polyps (**a**). The use of virtual chromoendoscopy with iScan 2 (enhancement plus surface enhancement tone) enhances minute changes of the mucosa and vascular structures, with better identification of ulcerations and characterization of pseudo polyps (**b**)

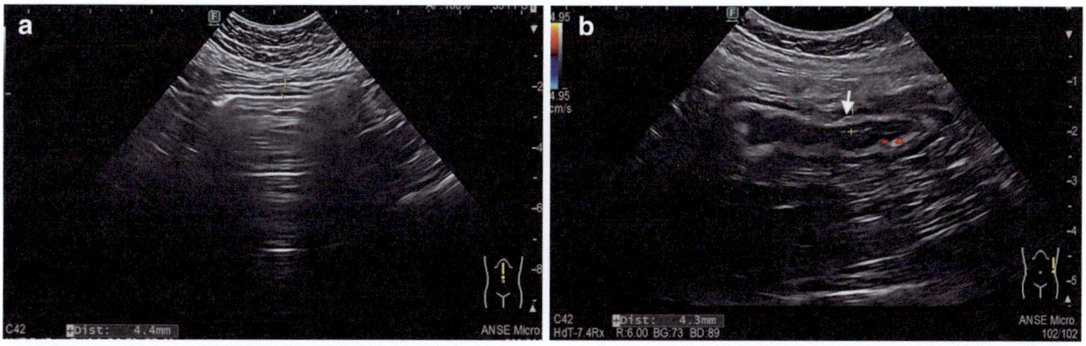

Fig. 6.3 Intestinal ultrasound. The transverse colon has mild wall thickening with normal echo pattern but thickening of the submucosa (**a**), while the descending colon has wall thickening with focal alterations of the submucosa (**b**, white arrow) and increased vascularization (Limberg score 2/4)

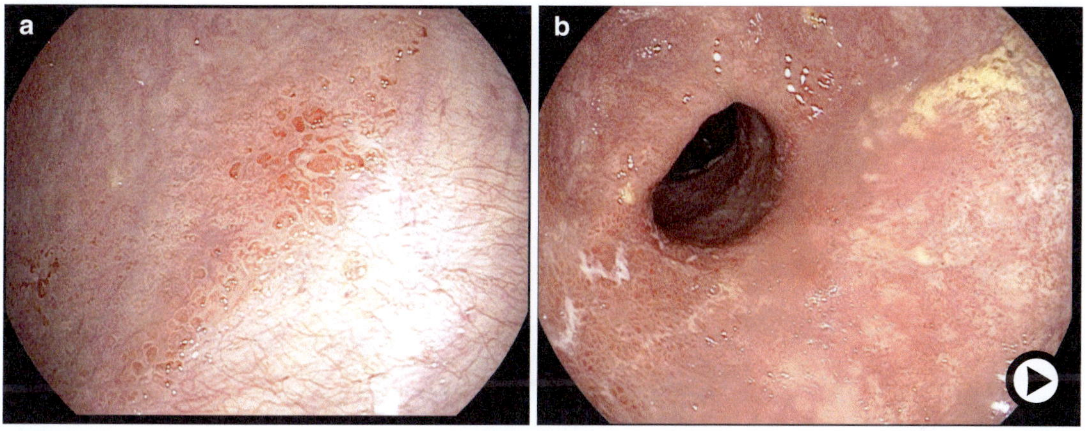

Fig. 6.4 Endoscopy. Focal hyperemia of the mucosa in the transverse colon (**a**); hyperemia with erosion and linear ulcerations in the descending colon, just after splenic flexure (**b**). Video description: Firstly, the terminal ileum is visible with normal bowel wall thickness and echo structure. In the right iliac fossa multiple reactive lymph nodes are present in the context of a fatty and hyperemic mesentery, near the cecum that appears distended by feces, thickened (6 mm). The transverse colon presents loss of haustration and mild thickening of the bowel wall (3.2 mm); the parietal thickening of the descending colon is visible in a cross-sectional (6.4 mm) and longitudinal (4 mm) view, with increased vascularization (Limberg score 2/4). The sigma also appears thickened and vascularized (Limberg score 3/4) (▶ https://doi.org/10.1007/000-j2j)

6.2 Case 2

A 51-year-old man with ulcerative pancolitis since February 2023, treated with mesalamine and two cycles of systemic steroid (Figs. 6.5 and 6.6). Evaluation of patient before (Figs. 6.5 and 6.6) and after treatment with mirikizumab (Figs. 6.7 and 6.8; video 6.7 and 6.8).

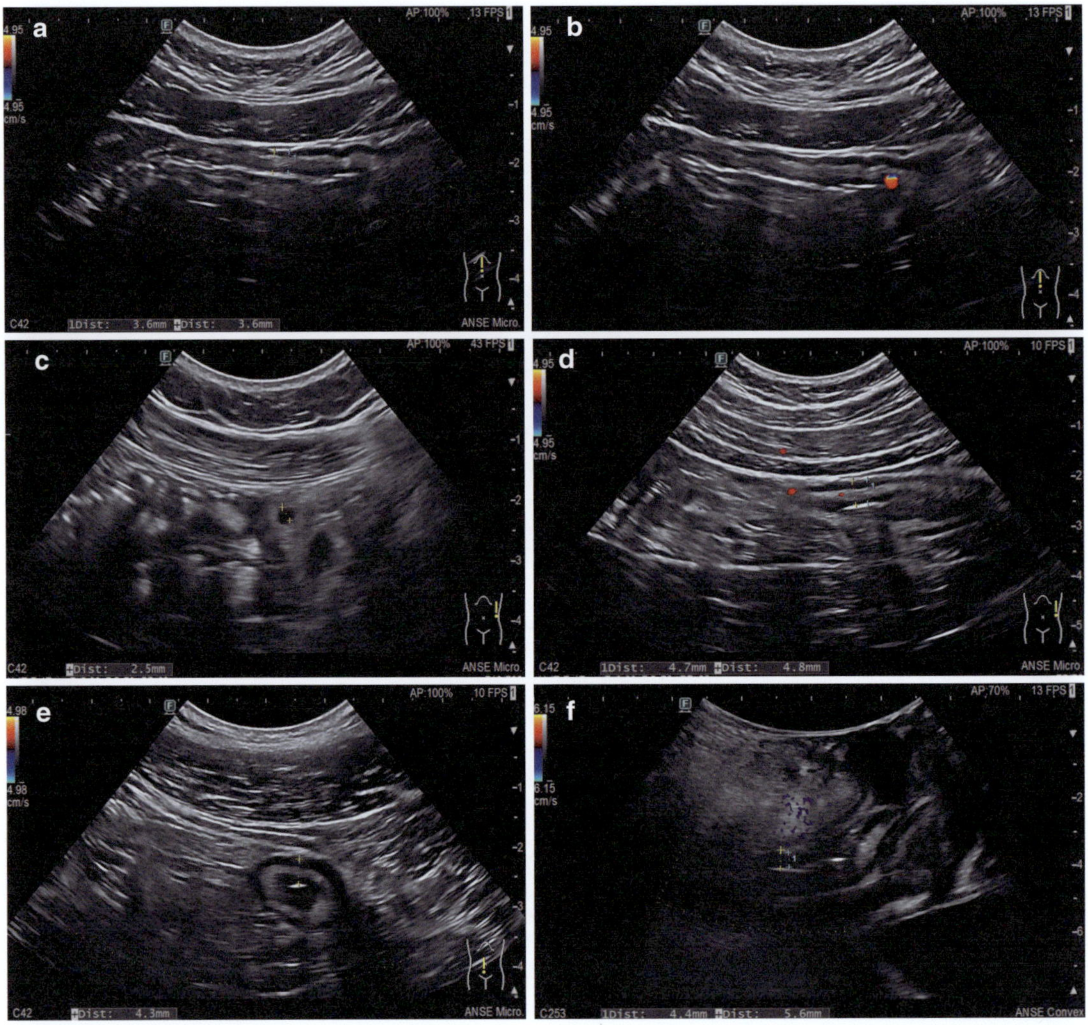

Fig. 6.5 Intestinal ultrasound before starting treatment with mirikizumab. The transverse colon has complete loss of haustration and is thickened with preserved echo structure but submucosa more prominent (**a**) and vascularized (Limberg score 2/4) (**b**). At the splenic flexure mesentery is hyperechogenic with reactive small lymph nodes (**c**). The descending colon has characteristics similar to those of the transverse colon (**d**). In the right iliac fossa, the distal part of the sigma can be seen in the cross section (**e**). Transperineal ultrasound shows longitudinal section of the rectal wall which is thickened up to 5.6 mm, with a predominantly hyperechogenic pattern (**f**)

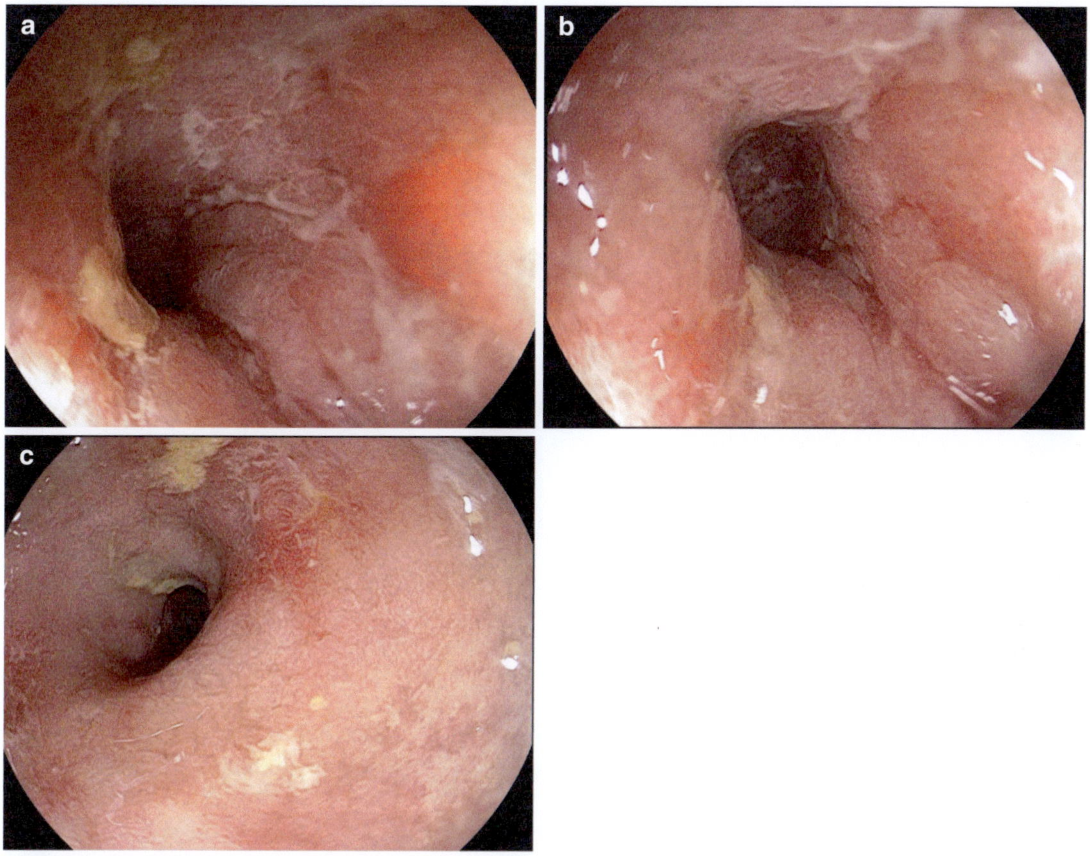

Fig. 6.6 Endoscopy before starting treatment with mirikizumab. The transverse colon has luminal narrowing, hyperemic mucosa with rarefaction of the vascular pattern, yellow spots, and presence of erosions and map-like ulcers (**a**). Similar characteristics can be seen in the descending colon (**b**). The proximal part of the ampulla of the rectum has a granular mucosa which is punctually hyperemic and covered with erosions and small ulcers (**c**)

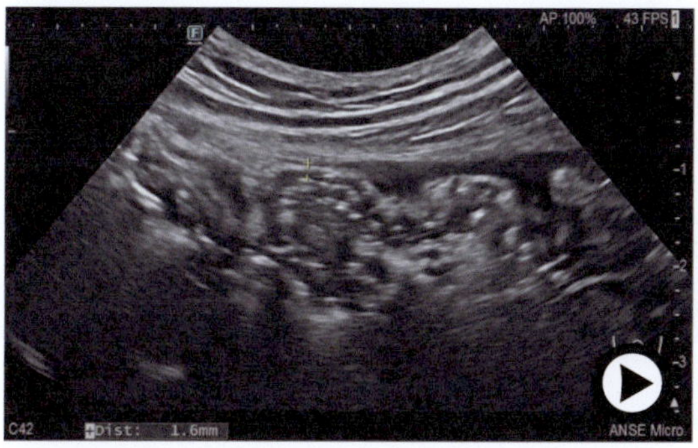

Fig. 6.7 Intestinal ultrasound after 8 weeks of treatment with mirikizumab. The distal part of the sigmoid colon has wall thickening, evident both in the cross section (4.3–4.7 mm) and longitudinal view (4–4.6 mm), with marked representation of the submucosa, which is vascularized (Limberg 2/4), and interruption of the mucosal layer due to the presence of ulcerations. The descending colon has similar characteristics (▶ https://doi.org/10.1007/000-j2g)

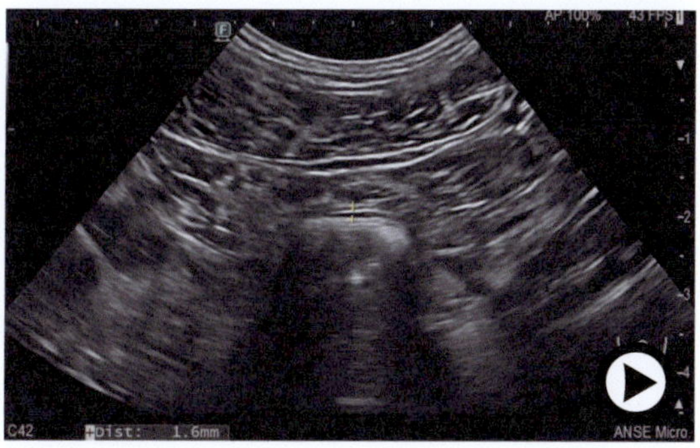

Fig. 6.8 Intestinal ultrasound after 8 weeks of treatment with mirikizumab. The transverse colon presents wall thickening (3.2–3.5 mm in the longitudinal section), vascularization (Limberg score 3/4), and multiple reactive lymph nodes in a fatty mesentery (▶ https://doi.org/10.1007/000-j2h)

6.3 Case 3

A 42-year-old man with ulcerative pancolitis since 2022, treated with mesalamine and multiple courses of systemic steroid. Evaluation of patient before (Figs. 6.9 and 6.10) and and after one year of treatment with infliximab and azathioprine (Figs. 6.11 and 6.12).

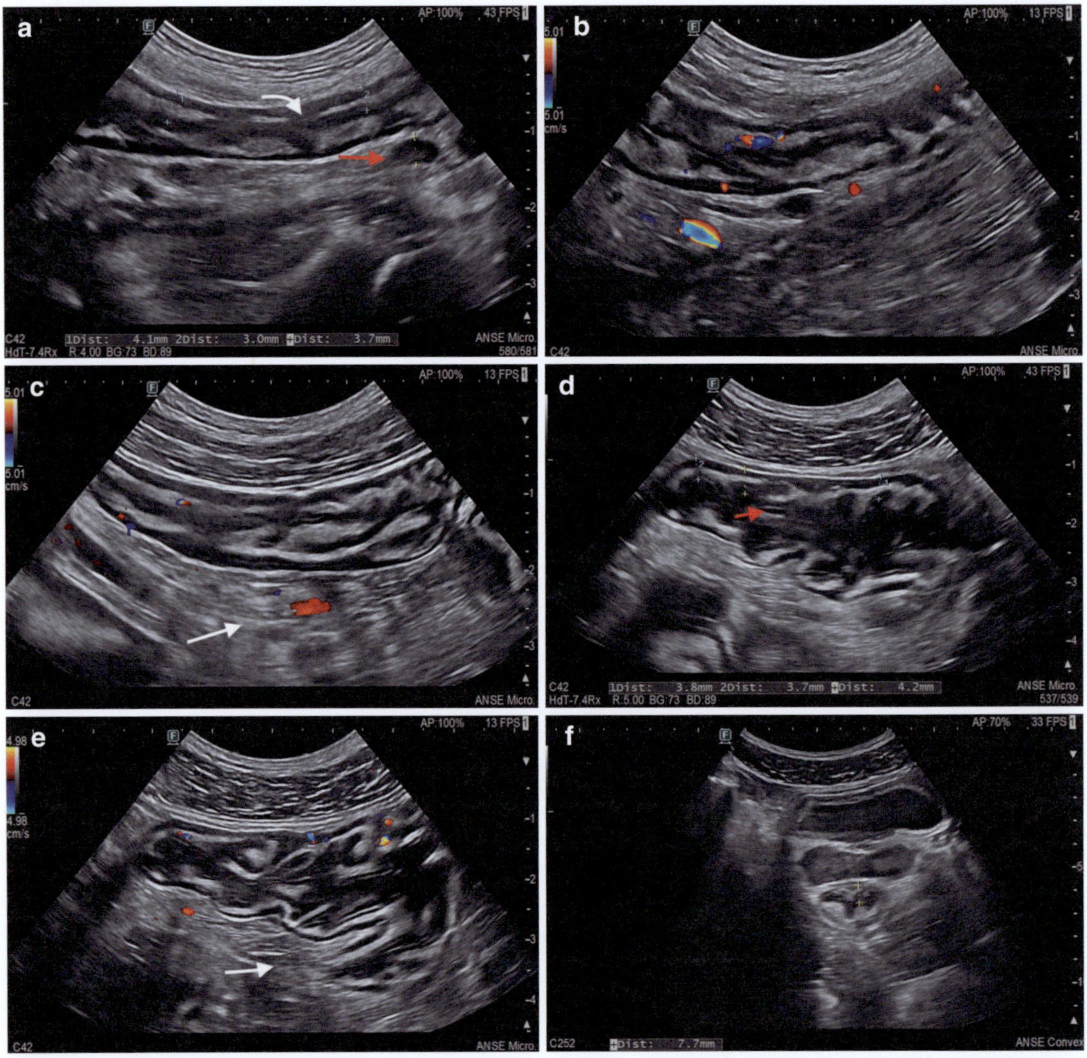

Fig. 6.9 Intestinal ultrasound endoscopy before starting treatment with infliximab and azathioprine. Thickening of the transverse colon with normal stratification but presence of focal alterations in the submucosa (white arrow) and adjacent reactive lymph nodes (red arrow) (**a**). Increased vascularization of the submucosa (Limberg score 3/4) in the same segment (**b**). Similar characteristics can be seen in the descending colon (**c**) which has increased vascularization of the submucosa (Limberg score 4/4), with adjacent mesenteric hypertrophy (white arrow). The sigma shows parietal thickening with regular stratification (**d**), narrowed lumen (red arrow) and increased vascularization (Limberg score 4/4) with adjacent mesenteric hypertrophy (white arrow) (**e**). The rectal wall appears thickened in cross-section (**f**) section on transperineal ultrasound

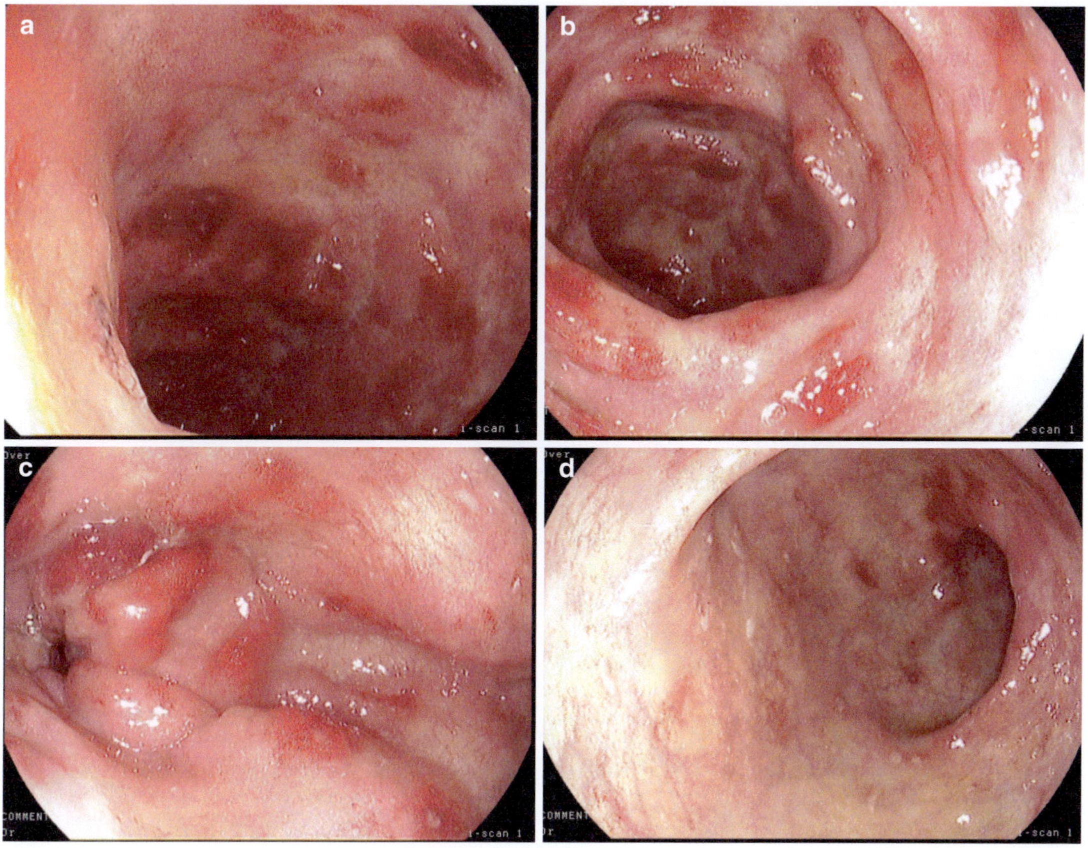

Fig. 6.10 Endoscopy before starting treatment with infliximab and azathioprine. Marked mucosal hyperemia of the transverse colon (**a**), descending colon (**b**) and sigmoid colon (**c**) with scattered erosions and reduction of normal haustration. The rectal ampulla is less hyperemic but shows rare erosions (**d**). The use of virtual chromoendoscopy (iScan 2) makes hyperemia and the presence of erosions more evident

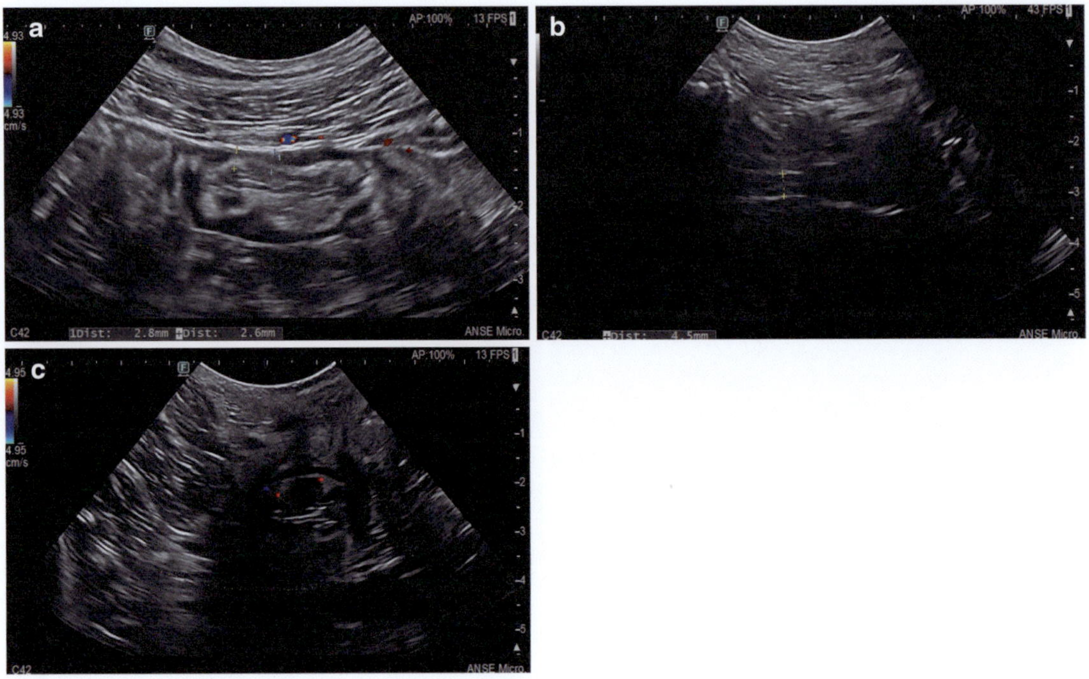

Fig. 6.11 Intestinal ultrasound endoscopy after 1 year of therapy with infliximab and azathioprine. The sigmoid has normal wall thickening and echo pattern without vascularization on color Doppler (**a**). On transperineal ultrasound, the rectal wall has thickness of 4.6 mm with preserved stratification in longitudinal section (**b**), with increased vascularization in cross-section (**c**)

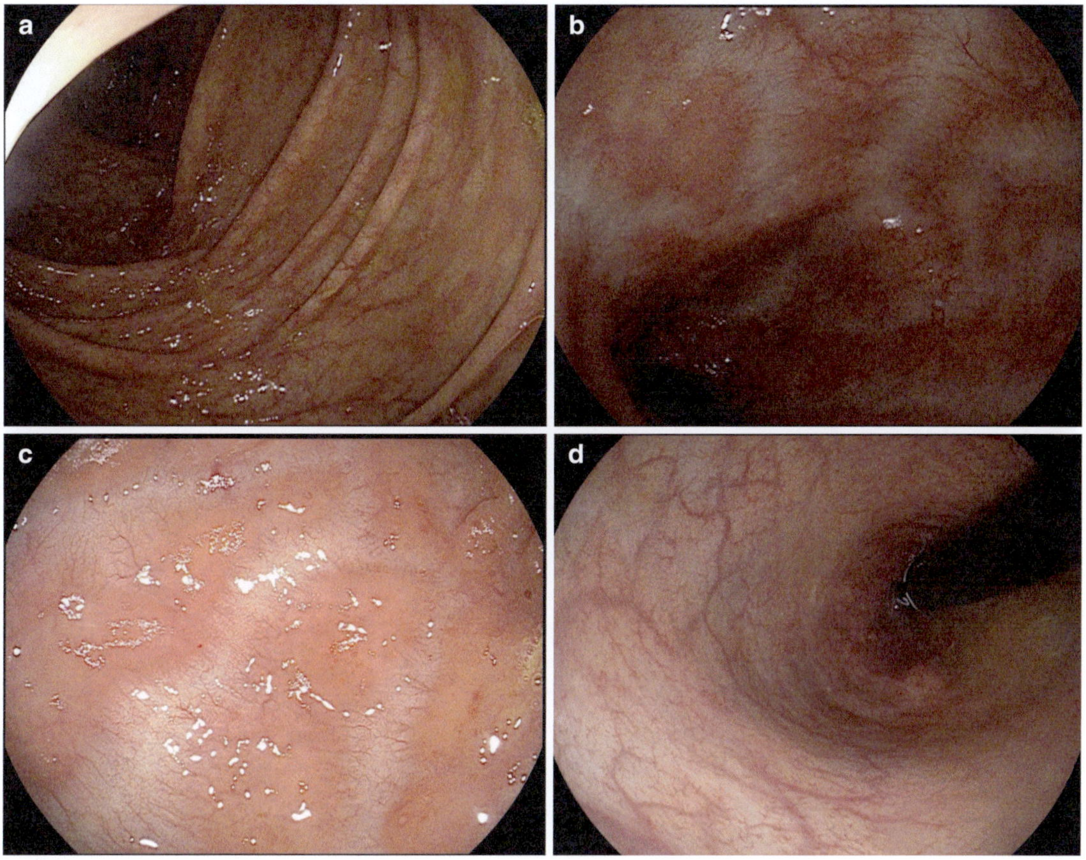

Fig. 6.12 Intestinal ultrasound endoscopy after 1 year of therapy with infliximab and azathioprine. The transverse colon has normal mucosa and haustration (**a**). The descending colon (**b**) and the sigma (**c**) show a slight reduction in the vascular pattern and some scarring. Slight mucosal hyperemia is seen in the rectal ampulla on retrospective examination (**d**)

6.4 Case 4

A 31-year-old woman with sub-total ulcerative pancolitis since 2019, treated with mesalamine and steroids, steroid dependent, started infliximab and azathioprine with clinical response and bowel ultrasound improvement (Figs. 6.13 and 6.14, Video 6.4).

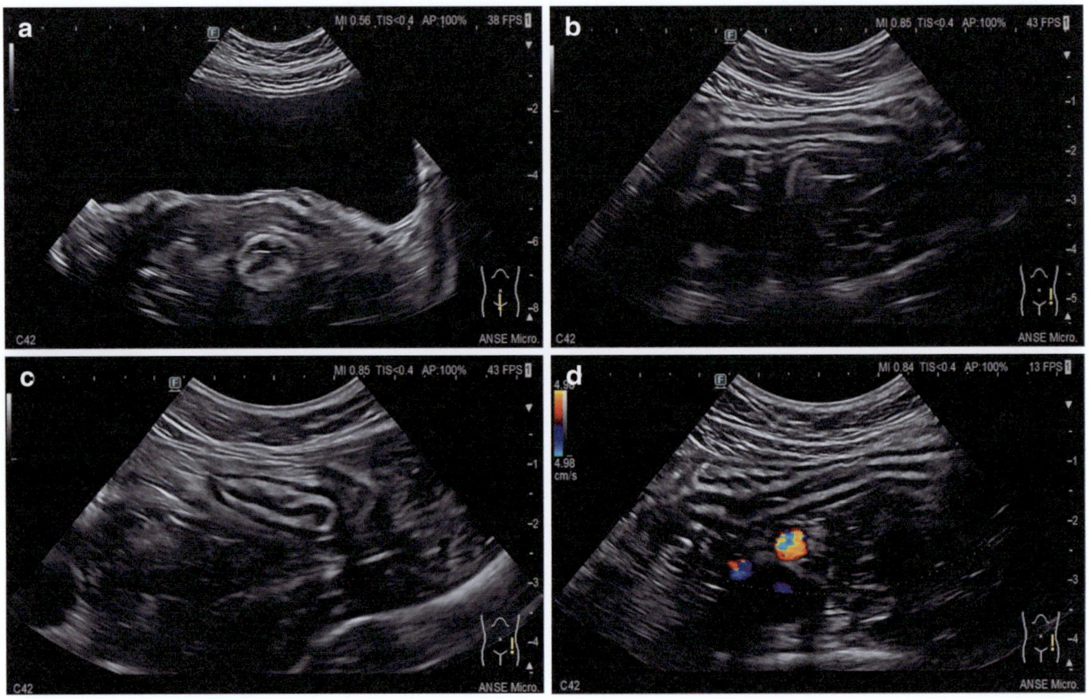

Fig. 6.13 Intestinal ultrasound before biologic treatment. Thickening of bowel wall in the rectum (**a**), sigmoid (**b** longitudinal, **c** transversal section) with normal stratification, submucosal layer well represented, regular vascularization at color Doppler (**d**) and regular haustration

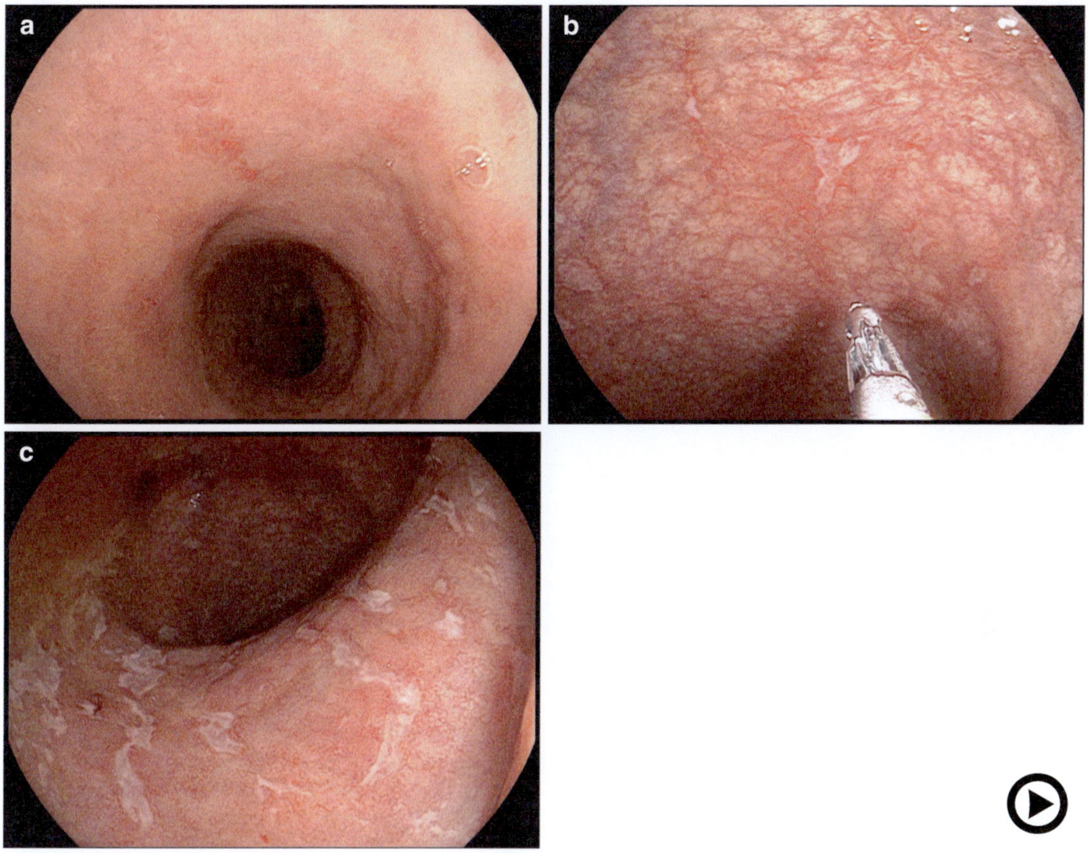

Fig. 6.14 Endoscopy before biologic treatment. The sigmoid appears hyperemic, fragile, and easily bleeding (**a**). In the rectum there are some ulcerations (**b**). Intestinal ultrasound evaluation after 8 weeks of treatment. Video desciption: The video initially shows the rectum with thickened walls and over-representation of the submucosal layer, then moving to the left iliac fossa we see the sigma also with stratified wall and over-representation of the submucosal layer, regular margins, no significant increase in vascularity on color Doppler. Wall thickness is normal (2.6 mm) after treatment (▶ https://doi.org/10.1007/000-j2f)

6.5 Case 5

A 76-year-old man with left-side ulcerative colitis since July 2022 and diverticular disease, treated with mesalamine and steroids, steroid dependent, started ustekinumab with clinical response and bowel ultrasound improvement (Figs. 6.15 and 6.16, Videos 6.5 and 6.6).

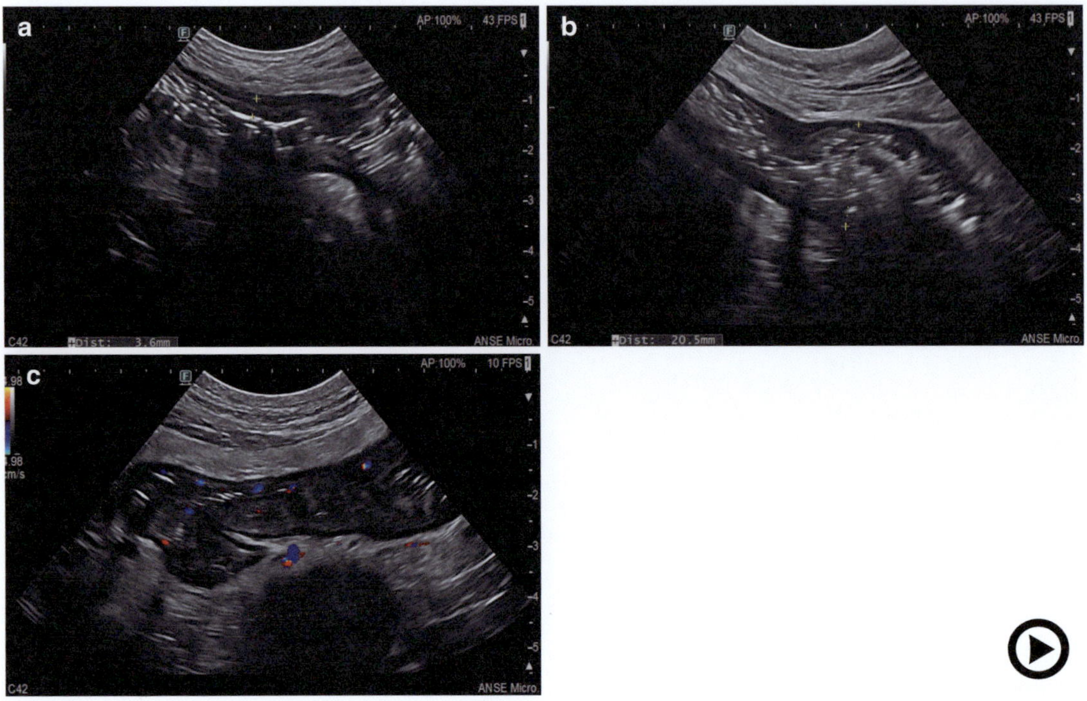

Fig. 6.15 Intestinal ultrasound before biologic treatment. Thickening of the bowel wall in the sigmoid colon in the longitudinal section (**a**) with attenuation of the normal stratification and retro-dilation of the descending colon (**b**). Increased vascularization (Limberg score 4) (**c**). The video shows a thickening of the walls of the sigmoid colon with alterations at the margins, indicating the presence of diverticula, along with increased vascularization observed with color Doppler (▶ https://doi.org/10.1007/000-j2k)

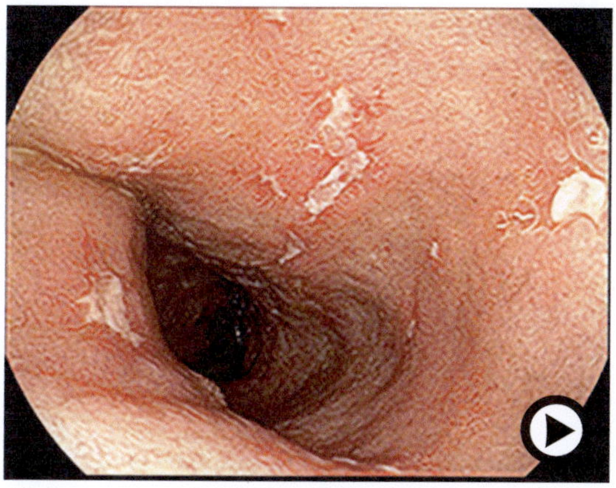

Fig. 6.16 Endoscopy before biologic treatment. The sigmoid appears hyperemic, fragile, and easily bleeding with some ulcers <15 mm. Intestinal ultrasound evaluation after 24 weeks of treatment. Starting from the hypogastric region, it is possible to visualize the bladder and the rectum. Moving to the left iliac fossa, the psoas muscle, iliac vessels, and the sigmoid colon can be seen, with walls of regular thickness containing gaseous and fecal material. Ascending along the descending colon, the walls appear regular and non-vascularized on color Doppler, with a thickness of 2.5 mm. Shifting the probe to the epigastric region, the stomach and adjacent transverse colon with regular walls, distended by feces and gas, are visualized. Finally, moving the probe to the right abdomen, the ascending colon, the psoas muscle, the iliac vessels, and the region of the ileocecal valve, all with walls of regular thickness, are visualized (▶ https://doi.org/10.1007/000-j2m)

References

1. Maaser C, Petersen F, Helwig U, Fischer I, Roessler A, Rath S, et al. Intestinal ultrasound for monitoring therapeutic response in patients with ulcerative colitis: results from the TRUST&UC study. Gut. 2020;69(9):1629–36. https://doi.org/10.1136/gutjnl-2019-319451.
2. Allocca M, Fiorino G, Bonovas S, Furfaro F, Gilardi D, Argollo M, et al. Accuracy of humanitas ultrasound criteria in assessing disease activity and severity in ulcerative colitis: a prospective study. J Crohns Colitis. 2018;12(12):1385–91. https://doi.org/10.1093/ecco-jcc/jjy107.
3. Allocca M, Filippi E, Costantino A, Bonovas S, Fiorino G, Furfaro F, et al. Milan ultrasound criteria are accurate in assessing disease activity in ulcerative colitis: external validation. United Eur Gastroenterol J. 2021;9(4):438–42. https://doi.org/10.1177/2050640620980203.
4. Allocca M, Dell'avalle C, Furfaro F, Zilli A, D'amico F, Peyrin-Biroulet L, et al. Early intestinal ultrasound predicts long-term endoscopic response to biologics in ulcerative colitis. J Crohns Colitis. 2023;17(10):1579–86. https://doi.org/10.1093/ecco-jcc/jjad071.
5. Allocca M, Dell'Avalle C, Craviotto V, Furfaro F, Zilli A, D'Amico F, et al. Predictive value of Milan ultrasound criteria in ulcerative colitis: a prospective observational cohort study. United Eur Gastroenterol J. 2022;10(2):190–7. https://doi.org/10.1002/ueg2.12206.
6. Sed NPO, Noviello D, Filippi E, Conforti F, Furfaro F, Fraquelli M, et al. Superior predictive value of transmural over endoscopic severity for colectomy risk in ulcerative colitis: a multicentre prospective cohort study. J Crohns Colitis. 2024;18(2):291–9. https://doi.org/10.1093/ecco-jcc/jjad152.

Role of IUS in the Differential Diagnosis with Other Colitis

7

Fulvia Terracciano, Chiara Lillo, and Spyros I. Siakavellas

7.1 Ischemic Colitis

Ischemic colitis is the most common form of ischemia affecting the intestinal organs. It is caused by a decrease in the blood flow to the colon, which results in a level of perfusion inadequate to support the vital functions of oxygen and nutrient delivery essential for cellular metabolism in the intestinal mucosa. The mechanism behind this seems to be most often occlusion of the mesenteric artery or generalized hypoperfusion of the mesenteric vasculature. Thus, it is more frequently seen in elderly patients, those with cardiovascular disease, and those who have undergone major surgeries. These patients represent a population with limited ability to regulate intestinal perfusion in cases of events affecting blood circulation in the area and subsequently are the ones most likely to exhibit this condition.

The majority of patients will have the transient form with spontaneous resolution of symptoms, but clinicians should be aware of the more severe form of the disease (about 15% of cases). This can result in gangrenous necrosis of the bowel wall, which can be life-threatening and requires quick recognition and appropriate action. There is also a smaller subset of patients that will exhibit a chronic form of the condition and develop long-standing complications such as strictures [1–4].

Diagnosis can be challenging as it usually concerns people with multiple comorbidities. There should be a high degree of suspicion in the presence of known risk factors such as constipation-causing medications and recreational drugs, conditions like immunosuppression, shock, major vascular occlusion, mechanical obstruction of circulation, and small vessel disease.

The clinical manifestations may be variable but usually include a rapid onset of abdominal pain and tenderness on palpation that corresponds to the affected area of the large intestine (usually in the left colon). Moreover, variable degrees of rectal bleeding may be observed, typically after the onset of the abdominal pain. Endoscopy is useful for identifying damage to the colonic mucosa associated with the condition but may

Supplementary Information The online version contains supplementary material available at https://doi.org/10.1007/978-3-032-11418-1_7. The videos can be accessed individually by clicking the DOI link in the accompanying figure caption or by scanning this link with the SN More Media App.

F. Terracciano (✉) · C. Lillo
Division of Gastroenterology and Digestive Endoscopy, Fondazione IRCCS "Casa Sollievo della Sofferenza", San Giovanni Rotondo, Italy

S. I. Siakavellas
Hepatogastroenterology Unit, 2nd Department of Internal Medicine, National and Kapodistrian University of Athens Medical School, Hippocration General Hospital of Athens, Athens, Greece

F. Terracciano et al. (eds.), *Bowel Ultrasound Compared with Endoscopy*,
https://doi.org/10.1007/978-3-032-11418-1_7

not always be available or even safe, especially in older and frail patients.

Computed tomography (CT) of the abdomen may be helpful to rule out additional causes of lower abdominal pain, but there is increasing evidence that point-of-care intestinal ultrasound may aid in the diagnosis in a similar and more timely manner [5–11].

7.1.1 Ultrasound Findings

Bowel Wall Thickening and Loss of Stratification

Ischemic colitis commonly presents with a diffuse or segmental thickening of the bowel wall (usually >5 mm). This can be seen on standard gray-scale ultrasound and is often more pronounced in the affected regions. It is usually more prominent than the thickening seen in inflammatory bowel disease but is comparable to the findings of infective colitis. Loss of stratification is predictive of severe ischemic colitis. Furthermore, the localized nature of the finding in a specific colonic area (usually longer than 10 cm) further orients towards ischemic colitis [7, 8, 12, 13]. Altered perienteric fat has been associated with severe transmural necrosis [14, 15] (Figs. 7.1, 7.2, and 7.3).

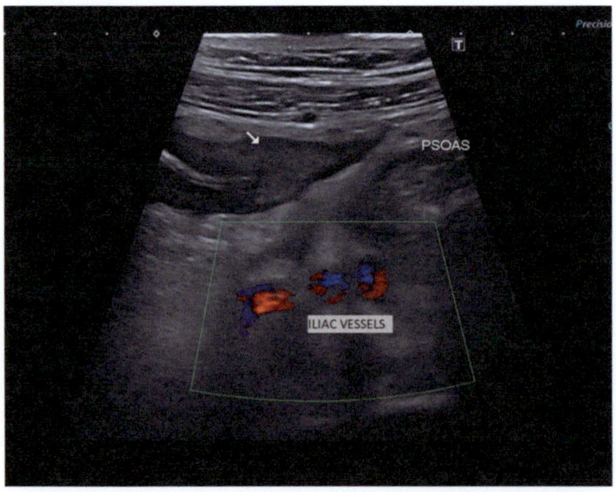

Fig. 7.1 In the picture, taken with linear probe, the arrow points to the sigmoid colon with thickened walls

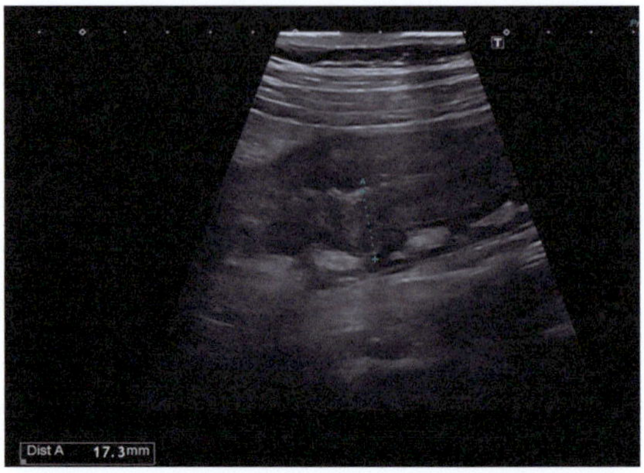

Fig. 7.2 In this longitudinal scan of the descending colon, a wall thickening of 17 mm is measured, along with hypoechogenicity of the mucosa and submucosa, which appear indistinguishable

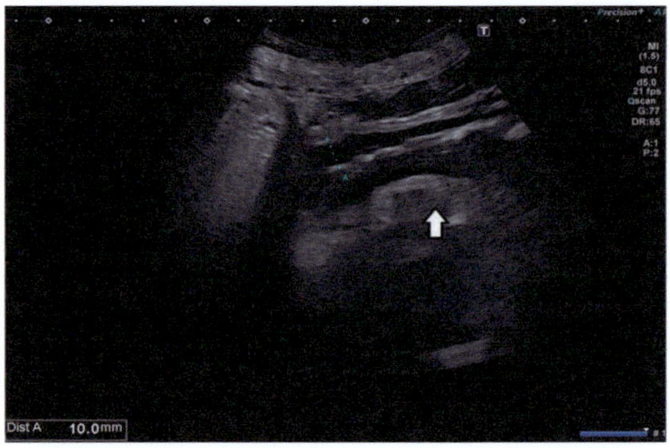

Fig. 7.3 In this scan of the sigmoid colon taken with a convex probe, the dashed line shows wall thickening with hypoechogenicity of the mucosa and submucosa. The arrow indicates thickening of the perienteric fat

Color Doppler Findings

Doppler ultrasonography may show diminished blood flow in the mesenteric vessels or in the affected colonic segment, supporting the diagnosis (Fig. 7.4) [13, 16–20]. Absence of mural flow is a hallmark sign of ischemia, but it may be seen only in 30–50% of cases [14]. CEUS may be used to assess perfusion in the bowel wall if there is any uncertainty in assessment with Doppler US.

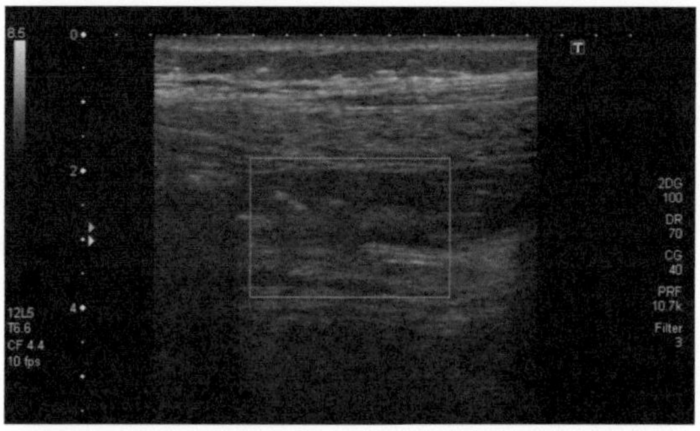

Fig. 7.4 In this scan with a linear probe of the descending colon affected by ischemic colitis, we can observe the absence of vascular signals

7.1.2 CT Findings in Ischemic Colitis [5, 9, 21, 22]

1. *Colonic Wall Thickening*
   - One of the most common and early findings: the colon may appear thickened, often in a segmental pattern, typically involving the left colon.
   - Thickening of the colon wall greater than 4–6 mm suggests ischemia, usually comparable to ultrasound findings (Fig. 7.5).
2. *Fat Stranding*
   - Increased density in the pericolonic fat (fat stranding) may be seen around the affected colon, indicating inflammation.
3. *Mesenteric Vessel Abnormalities*
   - In cases of arterial ischemia, there may be evidence of narrowed or occluded mesenteric arteries, often due to emboli or thrombosis.
4. *Bowel Distension or Dilatation*
   - In severe ischemia, bowel segments may be distended with gas or fluid, particularly in more advanced stages of colonic injury.
5. *Pneumatosis Intestinalis*
   - In cases of bowel infarction or necrosis, CT may show air within the bowel wall (pneumatosis), suggesting a more severe ischemic event and possible bowel perforation (Fig. 7.6).
6. *Reduced or Absent Colonic Enhancing*
   - If ischemia is severe enough to compromise blood flow, the affected segment of the colon may show reduced or no contrast enhancement on post-contrast images.

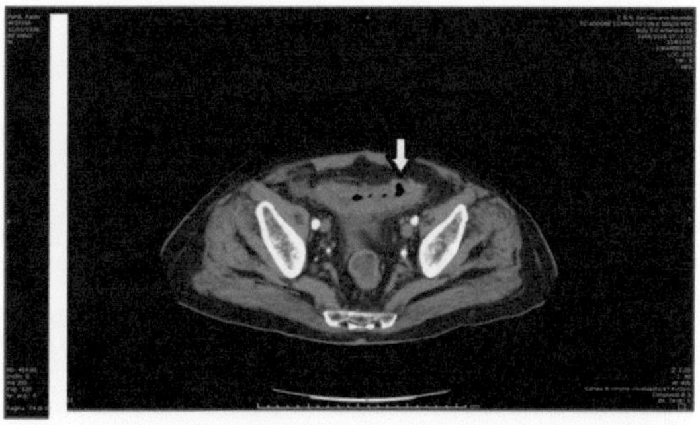

Fig. 7.5 In this CT cross-section, the arrow indicates a segment of the colon with thickened walls

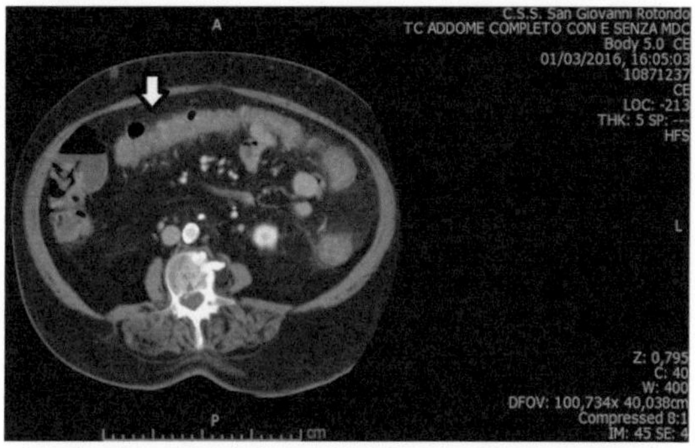

Fig. 7.6 In this CT cross-section, we see an example of a segment of the sigmoid colon with thickened walls and intestinal pneumatosis

7. *Absence of Colonic Haustration*
   - Loss of the normal haustral folds may be noted in ischemic regions of the colon [5].

7.1.3 Endoscopic Findings in Ischemic Colitis [23]

1. *Erythema and Mucosal Pallor*
   - The mucosa in ischemic areas may appear pale or dusky, reflecting reduced blood flow. In some cases, erythema (redness) can be observed due to inflammation (Fig. 7.7).
2. *Hemorrhagic or Bloody Lesions*
   - Superficial ulcerations or hemorrhagic spots may be visible, and mucosal bleed-

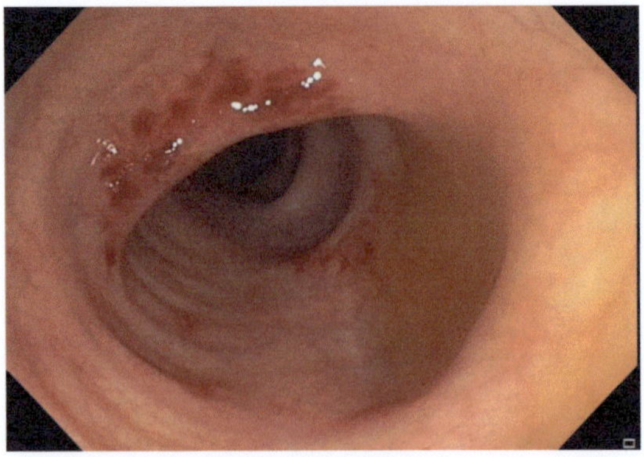

Fig. 7.7 The endoscopic image shows a segment of pale colonic mucosa with some erythematous areas at the apex of the folds

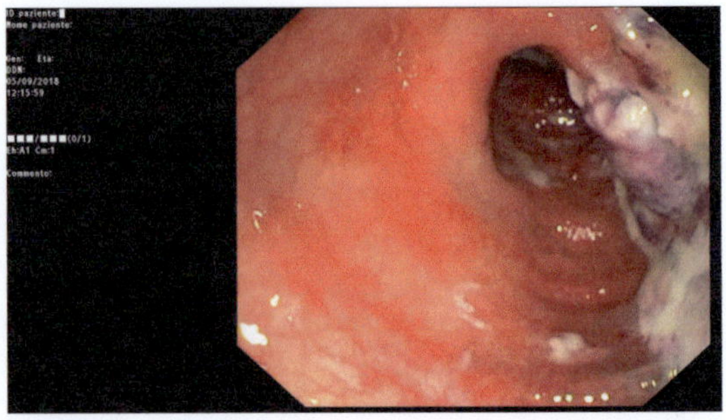

Fig. 7.8 In this endoscopic image, we can observe pallor and erythema of the descending colon mucosa, and on the right, ulcerated and necrotic lesions that typically develop on only one side of the wall

ing is often evident during the procedure. Larger lesions may result in frank bleeding.

3. *Segmental Involvement*
   - The affected areas often appear in a segmental, patchy distribution, frequently involving the left colon or sigmoid, while the rectum is typically spared.
4. *Ulceration or Necrosis*
   - In more advanced cases, endoscopy may reveal deep ulcerations, sloughing, and necrosis of the colonic mucosa. This typically occurs in more severe ischemic injury or infarction (Fig. 7.8).
5. *Bluish or Cyanotic Mucosa*
   - The mucosa in severely ischemic areas may have a bluish color due to hypoxia.
6. *Pseudomembranous Appearance*
   - In some cases, a pseudomembranous layer may develop over the ischemic mucosa, indicating significant injury and inflammation [22] (Fig. 7.9).

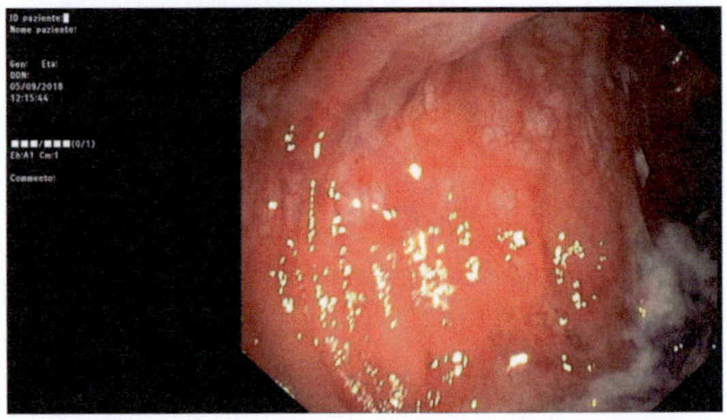

Fig. 7.9 Sometimes, ischemic lesions can be covered by membranes that resemble pseudomembranous colitis

7.1.4 Clinical Relevance

When there is strong suspicion of ischemic colitis, an intestinal ultrasound study may be performed as a point-of-care option. This allows for the detection of signs suggestive of ischemic colitis and may also delineate the extent of the affected colonic area. Subsequently, rectosigmoidoscopy may be performed, if feasible and safe, to provide direct visualization of the mucosal damage. While ultrasound provides an initial assessment of ischemic colitis, further imaging modalities such as CT or MR angiography may be required to fully evaluate mesenteric ischemia and its extent [14].

Ultrasound and CT have a similar diagnostic performance in ischemic colitis, except for the detection of intestinal pneumatosis—a rare and late finding associated with a poor prognosis—which is easily identifiable on CT but difficult to detect with ultrasound.

7.2 Infective Colitis

Infective colitis refers to inflammation of the colon caused by a variety of microbial pathogens (bacterial, viral, or parasitic). While "infective colitis" is thus considered an umbrella term, there are some common symptoms in these cases such as fever, diarrhea, abdominal pain along with nausea and even vomiting. These may be localized or generalized and non-specific making the differential diagnosis from inflammatory bowel disease and appendicitis challenging.

Infectious colitis and gastroenteritis in general are one of the most common causes of morbidity worldwide, especially in the developing world. In immunocompetent adults this condition is usually self-limiting and of short duration as a healthy immune system can respond appropriately and energetically to infection. On the other hand, immunocompromised or people with either immature or dysfunctional immunity such as elderly and children may exhibit significant morbidity and mortality. Commonly identified pathogens include Yersinia, Campylobacter, Shigella, and Salmonella, while recently of particular concern is the increasing trend of pseudomembranous colitis infections due to *Clostridium difficile* (*C. difficile*) secondary to excessive antibiotic use.

Infection is usually spread by water or food contaminated by the microbe in question. A shorter or longer (6–48 hours commonly) incubation period follows and then the full blown clinical syndrome develops with cramping generalized or localized abdominal pain being the most prominent signs. The signs associated with colitis are most often not specific enough to pinpoint to a distinct microbe as its cause. The combination of pyrexia along with the presence of raised inflammatory markers (white cell count, C-reactive proteine, fecal calprotectin) may be sufficient to rule out a functional cause of the symptoms, but for a conclusive etiological diagnosis identification of the infective agent needs to be achieved in cultures or via serology.

The role of intestinal ultrasound in this category of disease is more limited. Nevertheless, it may be useful in providing a distinction between self-limiting infection and ruling out more severe and progressive conditions such as inflammatory bowel disease or appendicitis. Thus, it may be employed as a point-of-care technique in order to help in determining the next diagnostic or interventional steps in clinical management of a patient with a constellation of signs including abdominal pain, fever, and diarrhea.

7.2.1 Salmonellosis

Non-typhoidal Salmonella can cause gastroenteritis, leading to symptoms such as fever and diarrhea, which typically resolve within 3–7 days. In rare cases (less than 5%), particularly in vulnerable populations such as infants, the elderly, or immunocompromised individuals, the infection may lead to prolonged bacteremia or localized infections involving the abdominal cavity or nervous system.

Sonographic imaging of Salmonella enterocolitis often reveals thickening of the ileal and proximal colonic walls, sometimes accompanied by free peritoneal fluid or enlarged lymph nodes. In children, colonic wall thickening and ascites are commonly observed and correlate with markers such as C-reactive protein and stool occult blood. However, the prognostic value of these findings remains uncertain.

Salmonella enterocolitis can be distinguished from Rotavirus colitis based on the presence of ascites [24, 25]. Typhoid fever, caused by Salmonella typhi, typically presents with fever, abdominal pain, and a characteristic rash. Ultrasound findings in typhoid fever may include splenomegaly, thickening of the ileal and cecal walls, and enlarged mesenteric lymph nodes [26–30].

7.2.2 Shigellosis

Shigellosis, a primary cause of dysentery, presents with bloody diarrhea and is caused by different Shigella species. It primarily affects the distal colon. Ultrasound findings may include diffuse colonic wall thickening and preservation of layered stratification, features that can help differentiate it from ischemic colitis [31].

7.2.3 Yersiniosis

Caused by Yersinia species, yersiniosis results in enteritis or enterocolitis, typically accompanied by abdominal pain, fever, and diarrhea. This infection can mimic appendicitis due to right-sided abdominal pain.

Ultrasound in the acute phase often shows thickened bowel walls and enlarged lymph nodes in the right iliac fossa. In some cases, coalescent lymph nodes may form an abscess or show signs of necrosis [32–35]. Ultrasound is valuable for differentiating yersiniosis from appendicitis and for detecting complications such as liver abscesses in severe cases [36, 37].

7.2.4 Infectious Ileocecitis

Infectious ileocecitis is an infection of the terminal ileum and cecum caused by Yersinia enterocolitica, Campylobacter jejuni, or Salmonella enteritidis. It shares clinical symptoms with acute appendicitis, including localized pain in the right lower abdomen, but typically lacks or has mild diarrhea. The tenderness is less severe, and acute phase reactants tend to be more elevated than in appendicitis. Due to these similarities, infectious ileocecitis can lead to unnecessary surgery for suspected appendicitis. At surgery, the appendix appears normal, but the ileum and cecum show thickening with enlarged mesenteric lymph nodes, although these signs can sometimes be subtle. Stool cultures are rarely taken due to the absence of significant diarrhea, leading to a delayed diagnosis.

Ultrasound is useful in identifying infectious ileocecitis, especially in cases where appendicitis is suspected. It can distinguish between infectious ileocolitis, Crohn's disease, and appendicitis by showing characteristic features such as thickened mucosa (and sometimes submucosa) of the ileum, cecum, and ascending colon, along with enlarged mesenteric lymphnodes [26, 30]. The thickened ileocecal valve may also be visible. In contrast, Crohn's disease typically involves more severe inflammation with thicker, non-compressible bowel walls and additional complications like abscesses or fistulas, none of which are seen in infectious ileocecitis. Therefore, when ultrasound suggests an infectious etiology, bacterial tests are essential to differentiate it from Crohn's disease.

7.2.5 Ultrasound Features

- *Bowel Wall Thickening*: The hallmark of infective colitis on ultrasound is bowel wall thickening, typically more localized but may be diffuse in severe cases. The wall can appear hypoechoic due to inflammatory edema. This thickening is usually symmetric and homogenous in the affected area, while the presence of moderately to grossly enlarged regional mesenteric lymph nodes may be also commonly observed [14] (Figs. 7.10 and 7.11).
- *Increased Bowel Peristalsis*: Inflammatory processes associated with infection can lead to hyperperistalsis, visible on real-time imaging [14].
- *Abscess Formation*: In complicated cases, abscesses can appear as hypoechoic collections near the bowel wall although this finding is also commonly observed in Crohn's disease. Color Doppler can be helpful to identify vascularity within abscesses [14].
- *Ascites*: In severe cases we can find peritoneal fluid [36].
- *Enlarged Lymph nodes*: Mesenteric lymph nodes are located anterior to the right psoas muscle in the majority of cases, or in the small bowel mesentery [26, 32] (Fig. 7.12).

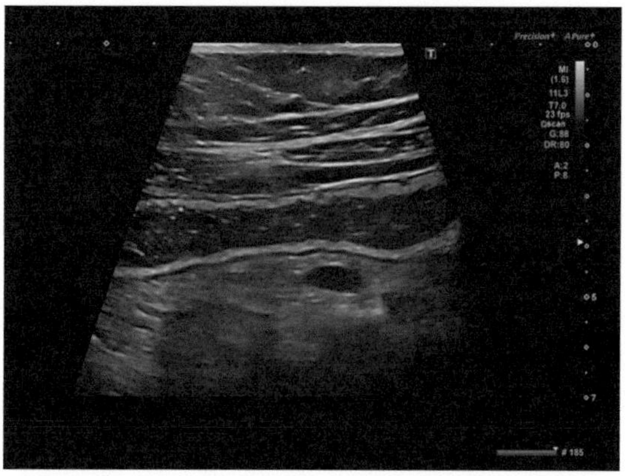

Fig. 7.10 In this linear probe scan of the transverse colon, we can observe wall thickening with a predominance of the mucosal layer, which appears hypoechoic due to edema, and an increase in liquid content typical of infectious colitis. Under the bowel we can notice an enlarged lymph node

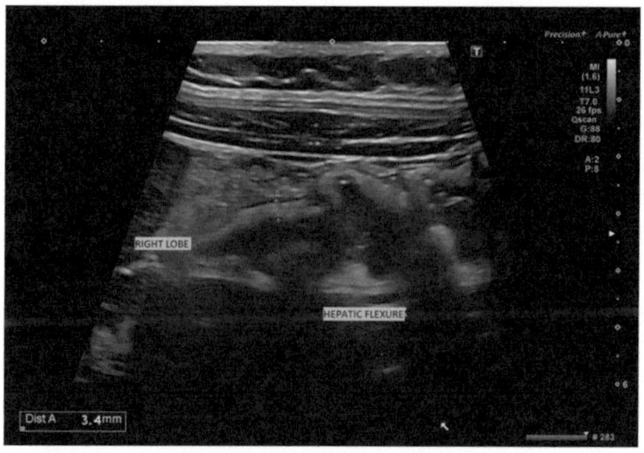

Fig. 7.11 In this scan, the right flexure of the colon is noted, characterized by thickening of the wall, which is homogeneous and symmetric, as well as an increase in the liquid content

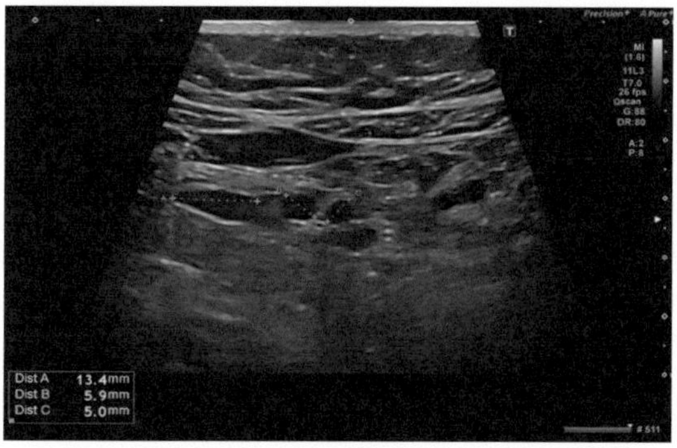

Fig. 7.12 In this scan, mesenteric lymph nodes with enlarged volume are measured. The lymph nodes are typically oval, hypoechoic, with a preserved hilum

7.2.6 CT Features [27, 37]

- *Bowel Wall Thickening*: Thickened walls (7–10 mm).
- *Enlarged Mesenteric Lymph Nodes*: Lymph nodes, typically oval or round, are often seen in the right iliac fossa, with a diameter not exceeding 2.5 cm. Lymph nodes may coalesce into an abscess in severe cases.
- *Hypodense Mesenteric Fat*: The fat surrounding the bowel may show hypodensity due to inflammation.
- *Abscess Formation*: In severe cases, abscesses or necrosis in the mesenteric region can be seen, indicating advanced disease.
- *Mild Free Peritoneal Fluid*: A small amount of free fluid in the abdomen may be noted in severe cases.

7.2.7 Endoscopic Features [38]

- *Mucosal Inflammation*: Characterized by mucosal erythema, swelling, and irregularity.
- *Ulcerations and Erosions*: Shallow ulcers or erosion might be visible.
- *No Strictures or Fistulas*: Unlike Crohn's disease, the bowel wall is compressible, and no stricture formation or fistulas are observed.

7.2.8 Pseudomembranous Colitis

Pseudomembranous colitis (PMC) is a severe form of colitis, primarily affecting the colon but sometimes involving the small intestine. The condition is typically caused by *Clostridium difficile* (*C. difficile*), which proliferates due to the use of certain antibiotics (such as ampicillin, clindamycin, and cephalosporins). Other rare infectious agents like *Staphylococcus aureus* may also cause similar symptoms. In some cases, PMC can occur without *C. difficile* infection, often due to factors like ischemic colitis, intestinal surgery, mechanical obstruction, or chemotherapy. Risk factors include age over 60, previous surgery, and use of a nasogastric tube, and conditions like malignancies, immunosuppression, and severe cardiac or pulmonary disease increase the risk of developing PMC. Hospitalization in an Intensive Care Unit and anti-ulcer medication are also contributing factors. PMC typically presents with watery or bloody diarrhea, moderate fever, abdominal cramps, and leukocytosis. Severe cases can lead to electrolyte disturbances, dehydration, and even life-threatening complications like toxic megacolon or colon perforation. Hypoalbuminemia can occur due to the rapid loss of protein from the gastrointestinal tract, potentially resulting in anasarca (severe edema) [39–41]. Radiological imaging (such as sonography and CT scans) plays a crucial role in diagnosing PMC, particularly when symptoms like abdominal pain, fever, and leukocytosis occur, as these could signal acute conditions requiring urgent treatment. Imaging can also help assess the extent of the disease and identify complications such as toxic megacolon, ischemia, abscesses, or perforation once PMC is confirmed [39, 42]. *C. difficile* is a Gram-positive, spore-forming bacterium that is responsible for 15–20% of antibiotic-associated diarrhea cases. The bacteria produce two toxins (A and B), which disrupt the normal colonic flora, contributing to the development of PMC. The gold standard for detecting *C. difficile* is the stool cytotoxin assay [43].

Endoscopy and stool assays are the primary methods for diagnosing PMC. In some cases, radiological techniques such as sonography or CT scans are used when endoscopic findings are non-specific.

7.2.9 Ultrasound Features

- *Colonic Wall Thickening*: PMC is characterized by marked thickening of the colonic wall, typically ranging from 10 to 30 mm, with an average thickness of approximately 11 mm. This thickening is primarily due to edema of the haustral folds (the mucosal folds of the colon) (Fig. 7.13) [44, 45].

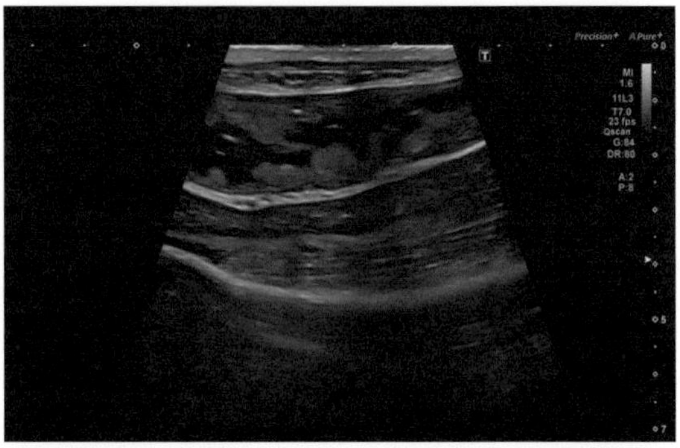

Fig. 7.13 In this scan with a linear probe of the transverse colon affected by *C. difficile*, we can observe the thickening of the wall, congestion of the submucosa, and the "accordion sign," which is an indicator of thickening of the colon folds

- *Accordion Sign*: A specific sonographic finding in PMC is the "*accordion sign*" or "*gyral pattern*," where the colonic wall shows characteristic folding [46, 47] (Fig. 7.13).
- *Submucosal Congestion*: The submucosal layer appears congested due to acute inflammation [46] (Fig. 7.13).
- *Reduced Mural Flow*: Decreased or absent blood flow is often seen in PMC, consistent with the inflammatory process [44, 45].
- *Ascites*: Present in 30–77% of PMC cases [44, 45] (Fig. 7.14).
- *Pericolic Fatty Tissue Infiltration*: In about 50% of PMC cases, infiltration of the pericolic fatty tissue is observed [45].

Ultrasound examination has demonstrated a sensitivity of 78% and a specificity of 94% for detecting PMC [48]. The most predictive findings include increased colonic wall thickness, hyperechoic thickening of the submucosa, and the presence of the accordion sign. However, features such as mural vascularization, pericolic fat changes, and ascites are less specific and less helpful in confirming the diagnosis of PMC. Ultrasound is particularly useful in the differential diagnosis between pseudomembranous colitis and other types of colitis (Table 7.1).

7.2.10 CT Features of Pseudomembranous Colitis (PMC) [39]

1. *Colonic Wall Thickening*
The most common finding in PMC is colonic wall thickening, typically greater than 5 mm. This thickening results from mucosal edema and inflammation. Wall thickness may range from 10 to 30 mm, with an average of approximately 11 mm. In severe cases, thickening can be even more pronounced.
2. *Accordion Sign*
The "accordion sign" is a classic CT finding in PMC. It refers to the thickened and edematous haustral folds folding in a manner resembling an accordion. This sign reflects significant edema of the haustra and is characteristic of PMC.
3. *Submucosal Edema and Mucosal Congestion*
CT imaging may reveal submucosal edema, causing the mucosal layers to appear hypodense or thickened. Mucosal congestion, indicative of acute inflammation, may also be evident.
4. *Loss of Colonic Haustration*
In severe cases, the normal haustral folds (the pouches of the colon) may become flattened or lost due to swelling and inflammation of the colonic wall. This results in a smooth, featureless appearance of the colon on CT.
5. *Presence of Mural Gas (Pneumatosis)*
Pneumatosis, or gas within the colonic wall, can occasionally be observed in severe PMC cases. This finding may suggest underlying ischemia and an increased risk of bowel perforation.
6. *Ascites*
Free fluid in the peritoneal cavity (ascites) can be visualized on CT, present in approximately 30–77% of PMC cases. The presence of ascites is often associated with more advanced disease or complications such as toxic megacolon.
7. *Pericolic Fat Stranding*
Inflammatory stranding of the pericolic fat may be observed around the colon. This fea-

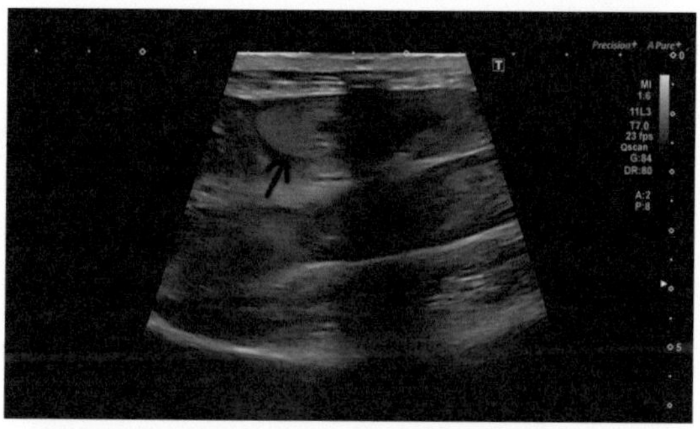

Fig. 7.14 A thin liquid film between the loops is present in 33–77% of cases of *C. difficile* colitis

Table 7.1 Differentiation of pseudomembranous colitis (PMC) from other colitis using ultrasound

Condition	Colonic wall thickness	Stratification	Mural flow	Accordion sign	Additional notes
Pseudomembranous colitis (PMC)	10–30 mm	Preserved	Absent or reduced mural flow	Present	Commonly affects the left colon, but can be diffuse
Crohn's disease	<13 mm	Preserved	Increased mural flow	Absent	Commonly affects the right colon
Ulcerative colitis	<9 mm	Preserved	Increased mural flow	Absent	Most commonly affects the left colon
Infectious colitis	<9 mm	Preserved	Present	Absent	Often involves the right colon
Ischemic colitis	11–12 mm	Loss of stratification	Absent in 60% of cases	Absent	Commonly affects the left colon, especially in severe cases
Colon cancer	>12 mm	Preservation in 20% of cases	Present	Absent	Limited extension of wall thickening, irregular pattern

ture indicates that inflammation is extending beyond the colonic wall into the adjacent fat tissue, a typical sign of acute inflammatory processes.

8. *Toxic Megacolon*
   In severe cases, toxic megacolon may develop, characterized by massive colonic dilation, with the transverse colon diameter exceeding 6 cm. This is a life-threatening complication that requires urgent medical intervention.
9. *Absence of Other Pathologies*
   CT imaging also plays a crucial role in ruling out other potential causes of the patient's symptoms, such as bowel perforation, intestinal obstruction, or ischemic colitis, which may present with similar clinical features.

CT imaging plays an important role in diagnosing pseudomembranous colitis (PMC), helping to identify characteristic features such as colonic wall thickening, the accordion sign, and the presence of ascites or pneumatosis. These CT features help in differentiating PMC from other types of colitis and guide appropriate management, especially in severe cases that may require urgent intervention.

7.2.11 Endoscopic Features of Pseudomembranous Colitis (PMC) [49]

1. *Pseudomembranes*
   The hallmark feature of PMC is the presence of pseudomembranes on the mucosal surface. These appear as yellow or white plaques that are raised and often loose or exudative in appearance. Pseudomembranes consist of fibrin, inflammatory cells, and necrotic tissue, and are typically found throughout the colon, especially in the distal colon and rectum.
   Pseudomembranes may be coalescent (fused together) or dispersed, with sizes ranging from small patches to larger, confluent areas.
   Lifting of the pseudomembrane: Upon gentle air insufflation or water irrigation during endoscopy, pseudomembranes may lift off the underlying mucosa. This is due to their typically loose adherence, in contrast to the firmly attached mucosal lesions seen in conditions like Crohn's disease or malignancy.
2. *Mucosal Erythema and Edema*
   In addition to pseudomembranes, there is often marked mucosal erythema (redness) and edema. The mucosa appears swollen, inflamed, shiny, and wet. Increased blood flow (hyperemia) is commonly observed, particularly around the pseudomembranes, contributing to a blushed appearance of the mucosa.
3. *Loss of Normal Mucosal Architecture*
   The normal haustral folds of the colon may become flattened or disrupted due to acute inflammation and mucosal swelling. Erosions and ulcerations can also occur as the inflammatory process breaks down the mucosal surface.
4. *Lack of Vascular Pattern*
   The normal vascular pattern of the colonic mucosa may be obscured due to severe edema and inflammation, making submucosal blood vessels difficult to visualize. This loss of vascular pattern is often a marker of significant mucosal injury.
5. *Focal or Diffuse Distribution*
   PMC can present with either focal or diffuse involvement of the colon. It is often more concentrated in the distal colon, particularly the sigmoid colon and rectum, although in severe cases, the entire colon may be affected.

7.2.12 Diagnostic Approach

Colonoscopy is the primary tool for diagnosing PMC. In some cases, flexible sigmoidoscopy may be sufficient, particularly when disease involvement is limited to the distal colon. The identification of pseudomembranes, along with associated mucosal edema and erythema, is usually sufficient to establish the diagnosis, especially when correlated with clinical features (such as recent antibiotic use) and microbiological testing (e.g., stool assays for *C. difficile* toxins).

7.3 Graft-Versus-Host Disease (GVHD)

Graft-versus-host disease (GVHD) is a serious complication following hematopoietic stem cell transplantation, affecting various organs, skin and liver above all, including the gastrointestinal tract. It can be divided into acute (occurring within 100 days after transplantation) and chronic [50]. The underlying mechanism of GVHD is an overt T-cell mediated immunologic response against the tissues of the recipient, which may lead to severe inflammation and damage. The bowel is one of the organs that can be affected by this reaction. Involvement of the gastrointestinal tract usually exhibits symptoms such as abdominal pain, diarrhea, and vomiting. The most prominent problem is ongoing diarrhea which can even lead to volume depletion. The combination of gastrointestinal symptoms with findings from other organ systems—such as a maculopapular rash on the palms and soles and hyperbilirubinemia—can aid in suspecting and establishing the diagnosis [51].

7.3.1 Ultrasound Findings

- *Bowel Wall Thickening*: Ultrasound typically shows diffuse bowel wall thickening, particularly in the ileocecal region which is most commonly affected, less frequently in small bowel segments. The appearance can range from mild to severe, depending on the stage and extent of the disease [52–54] (Figs. 7.15, 7.16, and 7.17; Video 7.1).
- *Motility* classified as hypoperistaltic, normoperistaltic, or hyperperistaltic [52, 53].
- *Color doppler imaging (CDI) Signs*: Bowel wall vascularity was graded as ischemic (no flow) or non-ischemic (normal or hypervascular). Additionally, the systolic and diastolic blood flow of the superior mesenteric artery (SMA) was evaluated to determine perfusion levels. Three categories of SMA perfusion have been identified: reduced, normal, and increased. Increased arterial perfusion of the bowel wall and SMA was common in most

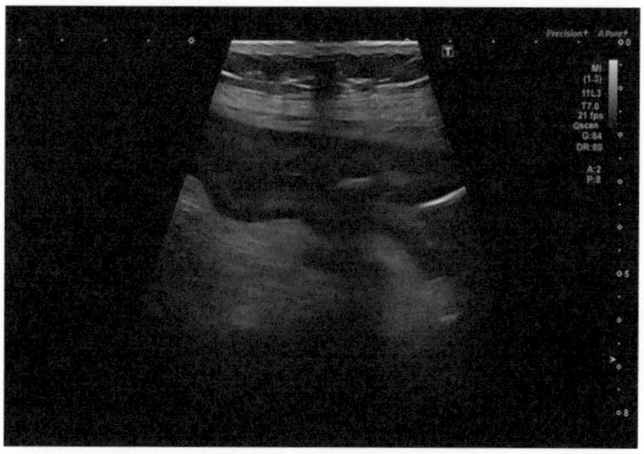

Fig. 7.15 In this scan using a linear probe of the descending colon in a patient with histologically confirmed GVHD, wall thickening and submucosal hypoechogenicity due to edema can be observed

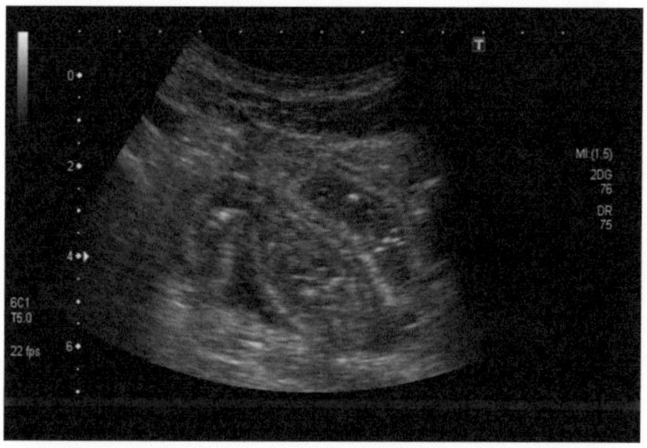

Fig. 7.16 More rarely, the thickening may involve the small intestine

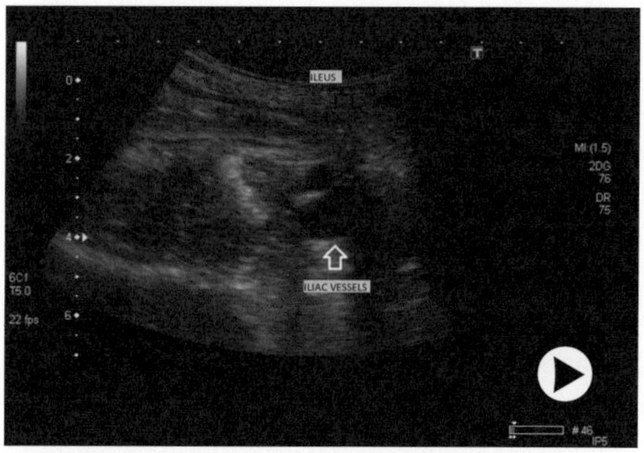

Fig. 7.17 The most frequently affected area in GVHD is the ileocecal region, as shown in this imageVideo 7.1 The most frequently affected area is the ileocecal region. The ileocecal valve and terminal ileum show thickness at the upper limits of normal, with mild hypertrophy of the surrounding mesentery and multiple reactive lymphadenopathies (▶ https://doi.org/10.1007/000-j2n)

patients with graft-versus-host disease, indicating an inflammatory process. However, some patients can have reduced SMA blood flow and ischemic bowel walls, showing a systolic velocity of less than 110 cm/s, with no diastolic flow. These patients have thickened bowel walls, but no visible blood vessels even with maximal sensitivity. The prognosis for these patients with ischemic bowel walls and reduced SMA blood flow was poor; they did not respond to immunosuppressive therapy and died within 2–5 weeks due to intestinal active GVHD. In contrast, patients with normal or increased blood flow responded to second- or third-line immunosuppressive treatments. Therefore, assessing SMA blood flow and bowel wall perfusion can serve as a prognostic marker in aGVHD [14].

- *Pneumatosis Intestinalis*: In advanced cases, pneumatosis intestinalis (gas within the bowel wall) may be visible. This finding indicates significant bowel ischemia and requires urgent attention [14].
- *Mesenteric Lymphadenopathy*: Enlarged mesenteric lymph nodes can often be seen in association with active GVHD [14].
- *CEUS Signs*: In a study by Schreyer et al. [55, 56], contrast-enhanced ultrasound (CEUS) was used to examine nine patients with histologically confirmed graft-versus-host disease (GVHD). The control group consisted of four healthy volunteers and six patients with Crohn's disease (CD). The study found that in six of the nine GVHD patients, the most significant bowel wall thickening was observed in the terminal ileum and cecum, with three patients showing involvement of the preterminal ileum. After administering 2.4 mL of SonoVue® intravenously, both GVHD and CD patients showed significant contrast uptake in the bowel wall. However, GVHD patients uniquely demonstrated transmural penetration of microbubbles into the bowel lumen, a contrast not observed in CD patients or healthy volunteers. The researchers concluded that the damaged gut mucosa in GVHD patients is more permeable, allowing microbubbles to pass through the mucosa and into the bowel lumen. They proposed that this penetration of microbubbles could be used as a novel diagnostic feature for GVHD, pending confirmation through controlled clinical trials.

7.3.2 CT Features [57, 58]

1. *Bowel Wall Thickening*
    - One of the most common findings on CT scans in intestinal GVHD is diffuse or segmental bowel wall thickening, particularly in the *small intestine* (especially the *terminal ileum* and *cecum*) and sometimes the *colon*. The thickening is typically *mild to moderate*, although it can be severe in advanced cases.
2. *Mucosal Edema*
    - CT may show *mucosal edema* in the affected bowel segments. This can be seen as an enhancement of the mucosa after the administration of contrast material.
3. *Pneumatosis Intestinalis*
    - Gas within the bowel wall (pneumatosis intestinalis) may be seen in severe cases, suggesting significant ischemia or necrosis of the bowel wall.
4. *Mesenteric Stranding*
    - *Mesenteric fat stranding* is a non-specific finding associated with inflammation and can be seen in intestinal GVHD.
5. *Ascites*
    - In more advanced cases, ascites may be present, which could result from severe bowel inflammation and increased permeability.
6. *Aneurysmal Dilatation*
    - Occasionally, *aneurysmal dilation* of affected bowel segments may be noted, reflecting significant damage to the blood vessels in the bowel.
7. *Hypervascularity*
    - Some patients may show *hypervascularity* on CT angiography, which can be indicative of inflammation and increased blood flow to the affected areas of the bowel.

7.3.3 Endoscopic Features [59]

1. *Bowel Wall Edema and Erythema*
   - *Endoscopic examination* may reveal *edematous* and *erythematous* mucosa, particularly in the ileocecal region and sometimes in the colon. The mucosa may appear swollen, red, and friable (easily bleeding).
2. *Ulceration and Necrosis*
   - Superficial *ulcerations* and *necrotic patches* are commonly seen in intestinal GVHD. These ulcers often appear *coarse* and *irregular*. In more severe cases, there may be *deep ulcerations*, with potential areas of necrotic tissue, indicating extensive mucosal damage.
3. *Loss of Vascular Pattern*
   - The typical *vascular pattern* seen on normal mucosa may be absent or indistinct due to edema and mucosal inflammation.
4. *Pseudomembranes*
   - In some cases, *pseudomembranes* or exudates may form on the mucosal surface, similar to those seen in inflammatory bowel diseases like *ulcerative colitis* or *Crohn's disease*.
5. *Stricture Formation*
   - *Fibrotic strictures* can develop in chronic cases of GVHD due to long-standing inflammation and scarring.
6. *Segmental Distribution*
   - Endoscopic findings tend to be *segmental* with involvement often restricted to particular regions of the intestine (e.g., terminal ileum, cecum, and ascending colon).
7. *Atrophy and Villous Blunting*: *Villous atrophy* and *blunting* may be observed under direct visualization, indicating chronic damage to the mucosal lining.
8. *Fistula Formation*
   - Rarely, chronic GVHD may lead to the formation of *fistulas* in the bowel, although this is more common in long-standing disease or after surgical intervention.

7.3.4 Clinical Relevance

Intestinal ultrasound monitors the progression of GVHD and detects complications such as bowel perforation or ischemia. Moreover, it may be used after transplantation to detect early signs of the condition. Thus it comprises an invaluable adjunct, bearing in mind, however, that the definitive diagnosis of GVHD relies on clinical, histological, and laboratory findings [14].

Ultrasound is also useful both for prognosis and for monitoring disease progression in cases of typhlitis, allowing early detection of complications as well as demonstration of improvement in milder courses. Given the complexity and severity of the underlying neoplastic disease in these patients it represents an excellent alternative to other imaging techniques and helps in obviating the need for endoscopic assessment.

References

1. Marston A, Pheils MT, Thomas ML, Morson BC. Ischaemic colitis. Gut. 1966;7:1–15.
2. Boley JS. Colonic ischemia-25 years later. Am J Gastroenterol. 1990;85:931–4.
3. Robert JH, Mentha G, Rohner A. Ischaemic colitis: two distinct patterns of severity. Gut. 1993;34:4–6.
4. Longo WE, Ward D, Vernava AM, Kaminski DL. Outcome of patients with total colonic ischemia. Dis Colon Rectum. 1997;40:1448–54.
5. Balthazar EJ, Yen BC, Gordon RB. Ischemic colitis: CT evaluation of 54 cases. Radiology. 1999;211:381–8.
6. Federle MP, Chun G, Jeffrey RB, Rayor R. Computed tomographic findings in bowel infarction. AJR Am J Roentgenol. 1984;142:91–5.
7. Jeffrey RB, Sommer G, Debatin JF. Color Doppler sonography of focal gastrointestinal lesions: initial clinical experience. J Ultrasound Med. 1994;13:473–8.
8. Bozkurt T, Richter F, Lux G. Ultrasonography as a primary diagnostic tool in patients with inflammatory disease and tumors of the small intestine and the large bowel. J Clin Ultrasound. 1994;22:85–91.
9. Philpotts LE, Heiken JP, Westcott MA, Gore RM. Colitis: use of CT findings in differential diagnosis. Radiology. 1994;190:445–9.

10. Ranschaert E, Verhille R, Marchal G, Rigauts H, Ponette E. Sonographic diagnosis of ischemic colitis. J Belge Radiol. 1994;77:166–8.
11. Chou CK. CT manifestations of bowel ischemia. AJR Am J Roentgenol. 2002;178:87–91.
12. Danse EM, Van Beers BE, Materne R. Small bowel wall changes in acute mesenteric ischemia: sonographic findings. Ultrasound Med Biol. 2000;26:A128.
13. Teefey SA, Roarke MC, Brink JA, et al. Bowel wall thickening; differentiation of inflammation from ischemia with color Doppler and duplex US. Radiology. 1996;198:547–51.
14. Maconi G, Bianchi Porro G. Ultrasound of the gastrointestinal tract, medical radiology. Diagn Imaging. 2013. Second Edition. Pages 71–74.
15. Hollerweger A, Maconi G, Ripolles T, Nylund K, Higginson A, Serra C, Dietrich CF, Dirks K, Gilja OH. Gastrointestinal ultrasound (GIUS) in intestinal emergencies – an EFSUMB position paper. Ultraschall Med. 2020;41(6):646–57.
16. Danse E. Imagerie des urgences abdominales non traumatiques de l'adulte. Encyclopédie Médico-Chirurgicale. 2004;33:705.
17. Quillin SP, Siegel MJ. Gastrointestinal inflammation in children: color Doppler ultrasonography. J Ultrasound Med. 1994;13:751–6.
18. Hata J, Haruma K, Suenaga K, et al. Ultrasonographic assessment of inflammatory bowel disease. Am J Gastroenterol. 1992;87:443–7.
19. Siegel MJ, Friedland JA, Hildebolt CF. Bowel wall thickening in children: differentiation with US. Radiology. 1997;203:631–5.
20. Shirahama M, Ishibashi H, Onohara S, Dohmen K, Miyamoto Y. Color Doppler ultrasound for the evaluation of bowel wall thickening. Br J Radiol. 1999;72:1164–9.
21. Horton KM, Corl FM, Fishman EK. CT evaluation of the colon: inflammatory disease. Radiographics. 2000;20:399–418.
22. Danse E, Dewit O, Goncette L, et al. Que faire en cas d'affection aiguë du colon? Une échographie, un scanner, des clichés conventionnels ou une endoscopie? SFR Paris octobre. Form Médica Contin. 2005;23:241–53.
23. Maimone A, De Ceglie A, Siersema PD, Baron TH, Conio M. Colon ischemia: a comprehensive review. Clin Res Hepatol Gastroenterol. 2021;45(6):101592.
24. Ueda D, Sato T, Yoshida M. Ultrasonographic assessment of Salmonella enterocolitis in children. Pediatr Radiol. 1999;29:469–71.
25. Bass D, Cordoba E, Dekker C, Schuind A, Cassady C. Intestinal imaging of children with acute rotavirus gastroenteritis. J Pediatr Gastroenterol Nutr. 2004;39:270–4.
26. Puylaert JMBC. Typhoid fever: diagnosis by ultrasonography. Am J Roentgenol. 1989;153:745–6.
27. Hennedige T, Bindl DS, Bhasin A, Venkatesh SK. Spectrum of imaging findings in Salmonella infections. AJR Am J Roentgenol. 2012;198:W534–9.
28. Mathis G, Metzler J. Sonography in salmonella enterocolitis. Ultraschall Med. 1992;13:106–9.
29. Mateen MA, Saleem S, Rao PC, Reddy PS, Reddy DN. Ultrasound in the diagnosis of typhoid fever. Indian J Pediatr. 2006;73:681–5.
30. Tarantino L, Giorgio A. Value of bowel ultrasonography in the diagnosis of typhoid fever. Eur J Ultrasound. 1997;5:77–83.
31. Fujii Y, Taniguchi N, Itoh K. Sonographic findings in Shigella colitis. J Clin Ultrasound. 2001;29:48–55.
32. Jelloul L, Frémond B, Dyon JF, Orme RL, Babut JM. Mesenteric adenitis caused by Yersinia pseudotuberculosis presenting as an abdominal mass. Eur J Pediatr Surg. 1997;7:180–3.
33. Matsumoto T, Iida M, Sakai T, Kimura Y, Fujishima M. Yersinia terminal ileitis: sonographic findings in eight patients. AJR Am J Roentgenol. 1991;156:965–7.
34. Pallister C, Rotstein OD. Yersinia enterocolitica as a cause of intra-abdominal abscess: the role of iron. Can J Surg. 2001;44:135–6.
35. Perdikogianni C, Galanakis E, Michalakis M, et al. Yersinia enterocolitica infection mimicking surgical conditions. Pediatr Surg Int. 2006;22:589–92.
36. Strungs I, Farrell DJ, Matar LD, Dekker L, Franz RJ. Multiple hepatic abscesses due to Yersinia enterocolitica. Pathology. 1995;27:374–7.
37. Leyman P, Baert AL, Marchal G, Fevery J. Ultrasound and CT of multifocal liver abscesses caused by Yersinia enterocolitica. J Comput Assist Tomogr. 1989;13:913–5.
38. Rutgeerts P, Geboes K, Ponette E, Coremans G, Vantrappen G. Acute infective colitis caused by endemic pathogens in western Europe: endoscopic features. Endoscopy. 1982;14(6):212–9.
39. Ros PR, Buetow PC, Pantograg-Brown L, Forsmark CE, Sobin LH. Pseudomembranous colitis. Radiology. 1996;198:1–9.
40. Cleary RK. Clostridium difficile-associated diarrhea and colitis. Dis Colon Rectum. 1998;41:1435–49.
41. Dallal RM, Harbrecht BG, Boujoukas AJ, et al. Fulminant clostridium difficile: an underappreciated and increasing cause of death and complications. Ann Surg. 2002;235:363–72.
42. Merine D, Fishman EK, Jones B. Pseudomembranous colitis: CT evaluation. J Comput Assist Tomogr. 1987;11:1017–20.
43. Kyne L, Warny M, Qamar A, Kelly CP. Asymptomatic carriage of Clostridium difficile and serum levels of IgG antibody against toxin. N Eng J Med. 2000;342:390–7.
44. Downey DB, Wilson SR. Pseudomembranous colitis: sonographic features. Radiology. 1991;180:61–4.

45. Truong M, Atri P, Bret P, et al. Sonographic appearance of benign and malignant conditions of the colon. AJR Am J Roentgenol. 1998;170:1451–5.
46. O'Malley ME, Wilson SR. US of gastrointestinal tract abnormalities with CT correlation. Radiographics. 2003;23:59–72.
47. Frisoli JK, Desser TS, Jeffrey RB. A sonographic sign of acute gastrointestinal abnormality representing submucosal oedema or haemorrhage. AJR Am J Roentgenol. 2000;175:1595–9.
48. Gallix B, Atri M, Bret P. Evaluation prospective de l'échographie haute résolution pour le diagnostic des colites pseudomembraneuses (CPM). J Radiol. 1997;78:S877.
49. Gebhard RL, Gerding DN, Olson MM, Peterson LR, McClain CJ, Ansel HJ, Shaw MJ, Schwartz ML. Clinical and endoscopic findings in patients early in the course of clostridium difficile-associated pseudomembranous colitis. Am J Med. 1985;78(1):45–8.
50. Filipovich AH, Weisdorf D, Pavletic S, et al. National Institutes of Health consensus development project on criteria for clinical trials in chronic graft-versus-host disease: I. Diagnosis and staging working group report. Biol Blood Marrow Transplant. 2005;11:945–56.
51. Mielcarek M, Martin PJ, Leisenring W, et al. Graft-versus-host disease after nonmyeloablative versus conventional hematopoietic stem cell transplantation. Blood. 2003;102:756–62.
52. Klein SA, Martin H, Schreiber-Dietrich D, et al. A new approach to evaluating intestinal acute graft-versus-host disease by transabdominal sonography and colour Doppler imaging. Br J Haematol. 2001;115:929–34.
53. Dietrich CF. Ultrasonography of the small and large intestine. In: Rose BD, editor. Up to date. Wellesley; 2010.
54. Haber HP, Schlegel PG, Dette S, Ruck P, Klingebiel T, Niethammer D. Intestinal acute graft-versus-host disease: findings on sonography. AJR Am J Roentgenol. 2000;174:118–20.
55. Schreyer AG, Landfried K, Zorger N, et al. Transmural penetration of intravenously applied microbubbles during contrast-enhanced ultrasound as a new diagnostic feature in patients with GVHD of the bowel. Bone Marrow Transplant. 2011;46:1006–11.
56. Piscaglia F, Nolsoe C, Dietrich CF, et al. The EFSUMB guidelines and recommendations on the clinical practice of contrast enhanced ultrasound (CEUS): update 2011 on non-hepatic applications. Ultraschall Med. 2012;33:33–59.
57. Kalantari BN, Mortele KJ, Cantisani V, et al. CT features with pathologic correlation of acute gastrointestinal graft-versus-host disease after bone marrow transplantation in adults. AJR Am J Roentgenol. 2003;181:1621–5.
58. Brodoefel H, Bethge W, Vogel M, et al. Early and late-onset acute GvHD following hematopoietic cell transplantation: CT features of gastrointestinal involvement with clinical and pathological correlation. Eur J Radiol. 2010;73:594–600.
59. Hiejima E, Nakase H, Matsuura M, Honzawa Y, Higuchi H, Saida S, Umeda K, Hiramatsu H, Adachi S, Izawa K, Kawai T, Yasumi T, Nishikomori R, Heike T. Diagnostic accuracy of endoscopic features of pediatric acute gastrointestinal graft-versus-host disease. Dig Endosc. 2016;28(5):548–55.

8 Transperineal Ultrasound

Giovanni Maconi, Antonella Marra,
Daniele Gridavilla, and Fulvia Terracciano

8.1 Introduction

Transperineal ultrasound (TPUS) is employed to assess the rectum and perianal area. This technique is characterized by its simplicity and non-invasiveness. It is a well-tolerated, universally accepted and low-cost examination, including in pediatric and neonatal patients. TPUS being a dynamic examination, it allows obtaining a multiplanar reconstruction of anorectal structures. Moreover, as a real-time method, it may be particularly useful in patients when endoanal ultrasound (EUS) and magnetic resonance imaging (MRI) are contraindicated or unavailable, and during follow-up visit for evaluation and monitoring of perianal disease. Thanks to the ability to integrate color Doppler and intravenous contrast-enhanced ultrasound (CEUS), it is possible to differentiate between phlegmons and abscesses [1].

8.2 Examination Position and Technique

The procedure does not necessitate specific preparatory measures for the patient. For reasons of hygiene the use of a probe cover is mandatory. Patients are typically positioned on their left lateral side with legs flexed at the knees (Sims' position) (Fig. 8.1, Video 8.1) [2]. To enhance anatomical visualization, it is advisable to have the urinary bladder moderately full. This technique is typically performed using standard probes, placed directly above the anus. Initially,

Supplementary Information The online version contains supplementary material available at https://doi.org/10.1007/978-3-032-11418-1_8. The videos can be accessed individually by clicking the DOI link in the accompanying figure caption or by scanning this link with the SN More Media App.

G. Maconi (✉)
Gastroenterology and Endoscopy Unit, ASST Fatebenefratelli-Sacco, Department of Biomedical and Clinical Sciences L. Sacco University Hospital, University of Milan, Milan, Italy
e-mail: giovanni.maconi@unimi.it

A. Marra
National Institute of Gastroenterology, IRCCS "Saverio de Bellis" Research Hospital, Castellana Grotte, Italy

D. Gridavilla
Gastroenterology and Endoscopy Unit, Fondazione IRCCS Casa Sollievo della Sofferenza, San Giovanni Rotondo, Italy

F. Terracciano
Division of Gastroenterology and Digestive Endoscopy, Fondazione IRCCS "Casa Sollievo della Sofferenza", San Giovanni Rotondo, Italy

F. Terracciano et al. (eds.), *Bowel Ultrasound Compared with Endoscopy*,
https://doi.org/10.1007/978-3-032-11418-1_8

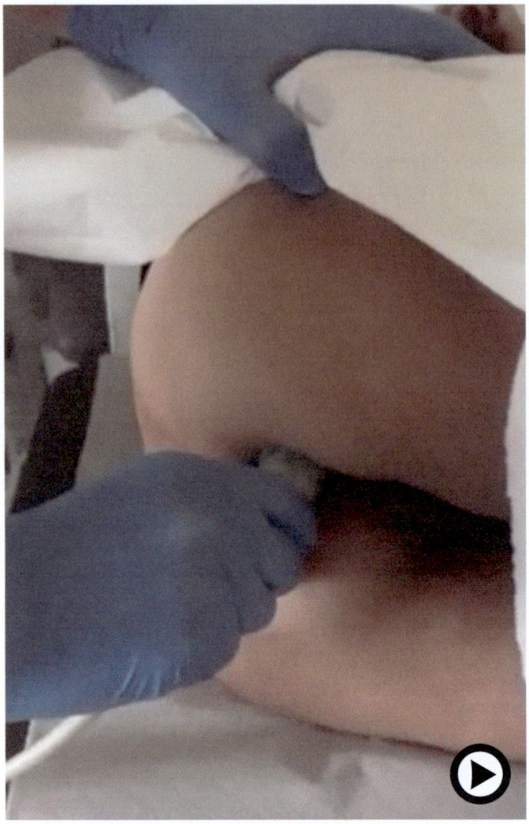

Fig. 8.1 Sims position. The probe is placed directly on the anus (▶ https://doi.org/10.1007/000-j2s)

conventional convex probes are employed, allowing for an imaging depth of 8–10 cm. The use of a microconvex probe is preferable due to its rotational capacity in the perianal area (Video 8.1). High-frequency (HF) linear probes are also useful for a better assessment of superficial structures in the perianal region and the perineum, especially those far from the anus.

8.3 Perineal Ultrasound Anatomy

Standard images are obtained through longitudinal and axial scanning above the anus, allowing the visualization of the anal canal, internal and external anal sphincters, the urinary bladder, and prostate or vagina. Depending on probe orientation, in the longitudinal scan it is possible to image the urinary bladder (with the anus on the top, positioned in the lower right side of the screen), the rectum (in the left quadrant), with a slightly oblique course (Fig. 8.2, Video 8.2). In this section, it is also possible to identify the anorectal angle (Fig. 8.3). In the coronal section the rectum is seen lower down, in continuity with the anal canal (Fig. 8.4, Video 8.4) Transverse scan-

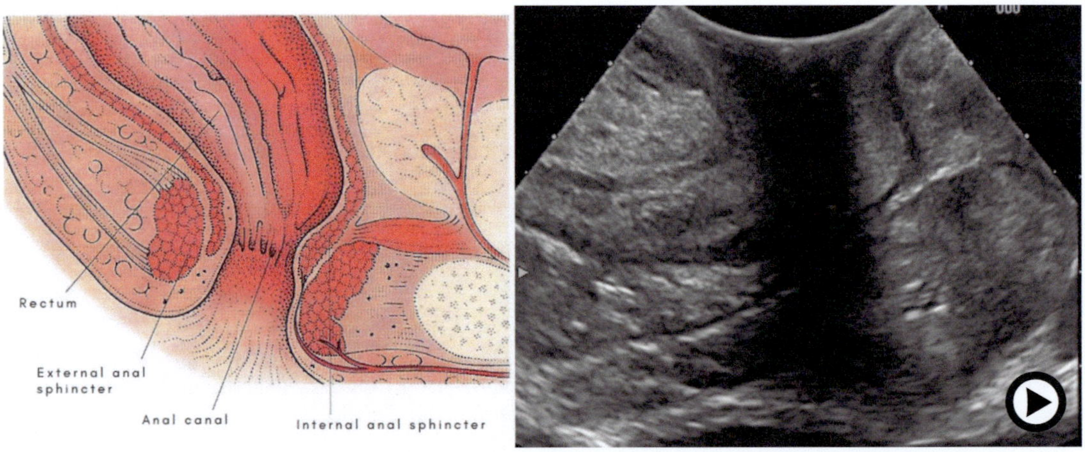

Fig. 8.2 Longitudinal scan of the anus. Anatomical representation of the anal region in the image on the left. The corresponding ultrasound image on the right (▶ https://doi.org/10.1007/000-j2q)

ning is achieved by positioning the probe anteriorly on the perineum, with the scan directed posteriorly towards the anus. This section is useful for identifying the internal opening of a fistula based on anatomo-topographical criteria according to the quadrants of a clock: anterior wall at 12 o'clock, posterior wall at 6 o'clock, left lateral wall at 3 o'clock, and right lateral wall at 9 o'clock. With this scan it is also possible to clearly image the internal anal sphincter (IAS), which appears as a thin circular hypoechoic band, approximately 3 mm thick. It is externally encircled by the external anal sphincter (EAS), which is a hyperechoic structure, slightly thicker than the internal sphincter. Its deeper part continues with the puborectalis muscle (Fig. 8.5, Video 8.5).

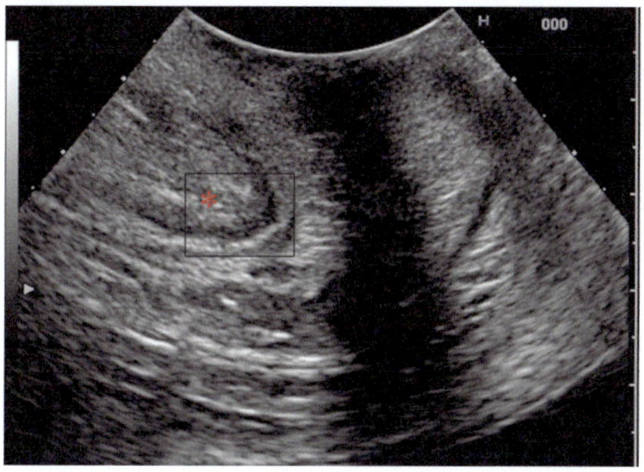

Fig. 8.3 In longitudinal scan the anorectal angle (*) is visible

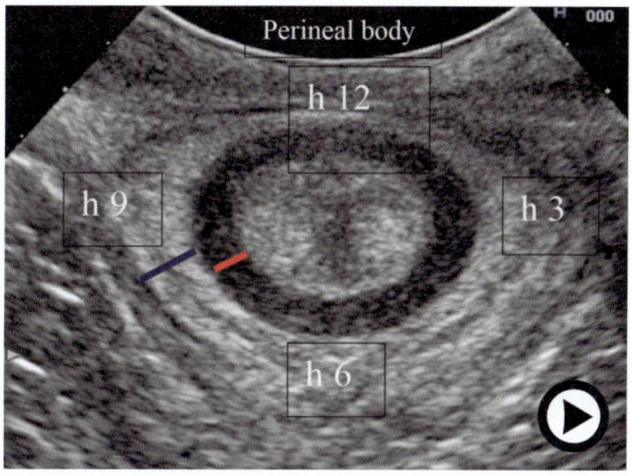

Fig. 8.5 Transversal scan of the anus with its perianal anatomical landmarks: *red line* internal anal sphincter, *blue line* external anal sphincter (▶ https://doi.org/10.1007/000-j2p)

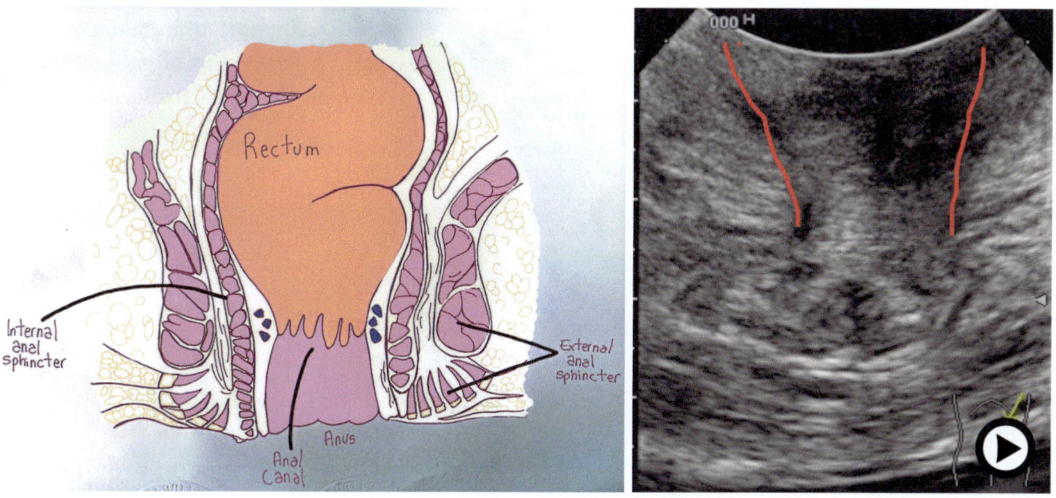

Fig. 8.4 Coronal scan of the anus. Anatomical representation of the anal region in the image on the left. The corresponding ultrasound image on the right (▶ https://doi.org/10.1007/000-j2r)

8.4 Perianal Fistulas and Abscesses

Transperineal ultrasound (TPUS) is an accurate method for diagnosing, classifying, and managing perianal fistulas and abscesses. These conditions are the main cause of perianal sepsis in patients with inflammatory bowel disease (IBD), particularly Crohn's disease [3].

A systematic review with meta-analysis showed that TPUS has high sensitivity in detecting perianal fistulas (98.3%) and their internal openings (90.6%) and in classifying fistulas (92.8%), and that it is also accurate in detecting perianal abscesses (sensitivity 86.1%, positive predictive value 88.4%) [4].

Perianal fistulas are typically characterized as abnormal communications that develop between the anus and the perianal skin, highlighted by continuous purulent discharge or recurrent episodes of swelling and tenderness in the perianal area.

Indeed, TPUS is often performed concurrently with a digital anorectal examination to first identify any areas of tenderness.

Fistulas are typically visualized as hypoechoic tracts, often containing gaseous artifacts, extending between the anus or rectum and the perianal surface or vagina. Typically, fistulas exhibit an irregular morphology, and may end blindly or form conncctions with other organs such as the uterus, urinary bladder, skin, or bowel (Fig. 8.6). The internal fistula opening is visualized as a hypoechoic area within the intersphincteric space, adjacent to the internal sphincter, and becomes more distinct when air bubbles are present.

Starting from the internal anal sphincter, the course of the fistula can be traced up to the perianal cutaneous opening, if present. The study of the fistula's tract can also be conducted by starting from the cutaneous orifice, following the fistulous tract to the internal opening. To enhance visualization of the fistula's course, its branches, and the internal opening, the injection of contrast agents (such as hydrogen peroxide or SonoVue) through the cutaneous orifice is useful [1] (Fig. 8.7).

An accurate classification of these lesions is mandatory for an appropriate management, often requiring a combination of medical and surgical therapy.

According to Park's classification, fistulas can be divided based on the location of the internal opening and their relationship with the sphincters into: superficial, inter-, trans-, extra- or suprasphincteric types (Fig. 8.8) [5].

Another classification based on anatomical and clinical parameters is the differentiation of fistulas as "simple" or "complex." Simple fistulas include superficial, low transsphincteric, and intersphincteric fistulas that cross <30% of the external sphincter. Complex fistulas include high

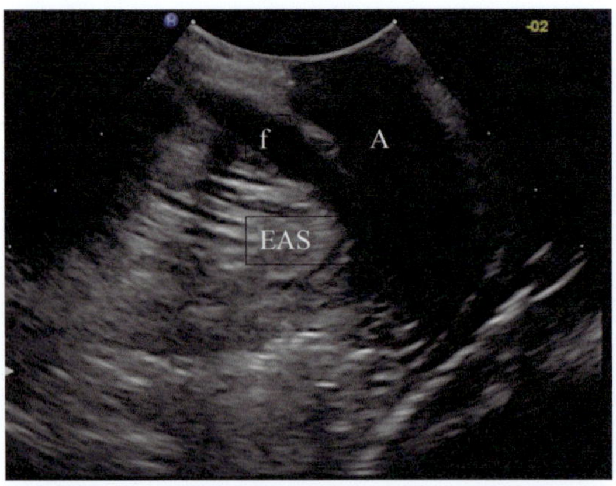

Fig. 8.6 Transsphincteric fistula appears as a hypoechoic tract that crosses the external sphincter. f = fistula, A = anus, EAS = external anal sphincter

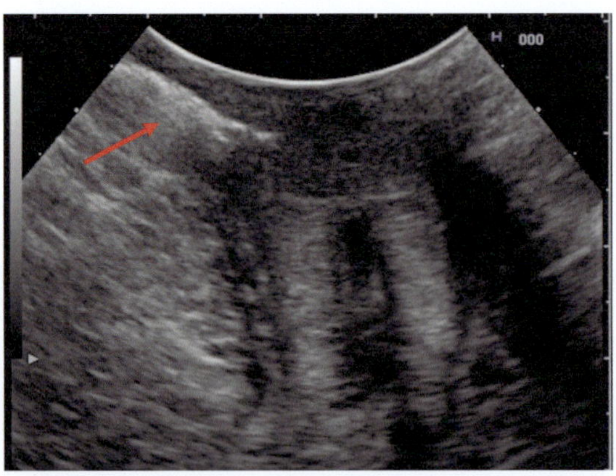

Fig. 8.7 Fistula is more easily detected after injecting of a contrast agent (such as diluted hydrogen peroxide) into the external opening. *Arrow*, contrast agent

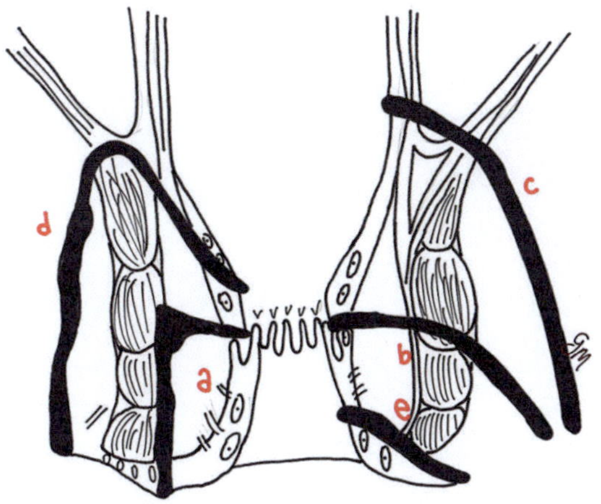

Fig. 8.8 Park's classification: (a) intersphincteric, (b) transsphincteric, (c) extrasphincteric, (d) suprasphincteric, and (e) superficial

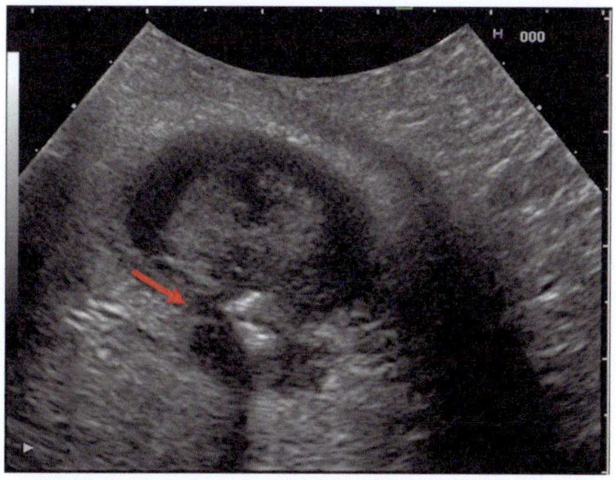

Fig. 8.9 Transversal scan of the anus showing an intersphicnteric fistula with internal opening at 6 o'clock. The fistula contains gas and is confined between internal and external sphincters

transsphincteric, suprasphincteric, and extrasphincteric fistulas, as well as horseshoe, recto-vaginal fistulas, and fistulas associated with abscesses or anal stricture [6].

Due to its restricted field of view and limited panormamic view, TPUS alone is insufficient for the evaluation of complex fistulas. In such cases, supplementary imaging techniques like EUS and MRI should be employed. In particular, MRI, due to its panoramic view, can also be more accurate in diagnosing complex fistulas [1].

Intersphincteric fistula appears as a hypoechoic tract running through the intersphincteric space, usually not exceeding 30% of the width of the external sphincter (Fig. 8.9). Transsphincteric fistula is visualized as a hypoechoic tract crossing the external anal sphincter. The transverse scan allows us to differentiate accurately (Fig. 8.10). These fistulas may develop ramifications or extensions, along the horizontal or cranial plane, called "horseshoe," that may be imaged by longitudinal scan as ovoid hypoechoic lesions just posterior to the anorectal junction or as a large curved hypoechoic area, posteriorly to the anus, in transverse scans.

Suprasphincteric and extrasphincteric fistulas typically do not cross the internal anal sphincter, originating at the anorectal junction or just above it. In addition to these types of fistulas, rectovaginal or anovulvar fistulas can be visualized as hypoechoic areas or tracts between rectum or anus and vagina or vulva (Fig. 8.11), while superficial fistulas are located distally to both the internal and the external anal sphincters.

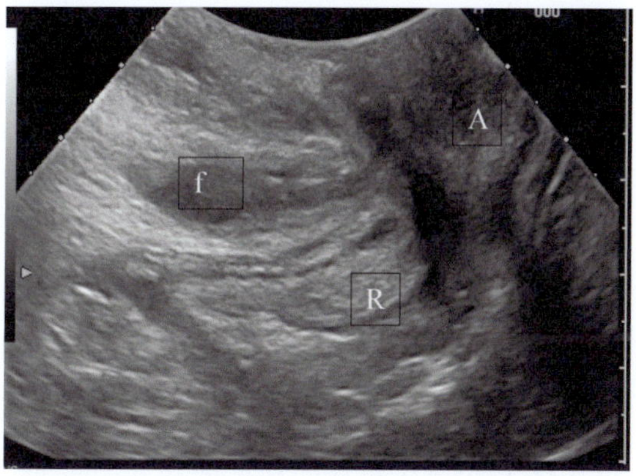

Fig. 8.10 Perianal sagittal scan showing perianal transsphincteric long sinus (blind-end fistula without external opening), arising posteriorly from the anorectal angle. The large diameter of the distal tract suggests a possible intermittent collection of material, and likely an abscess. F = fistula, A = anus, R = rectum

In complex fistulas, the first line of treatment is often a loose non-cutting seton. This option is safe and generally well-tolerated; it facilitates drainage of the sinus, and prevents the development of a more complex scenario. After placing a loose seton, anti-TNF therapy is typically provided as a subsequent treatment option (Fig. 8.12, Video 8.12).

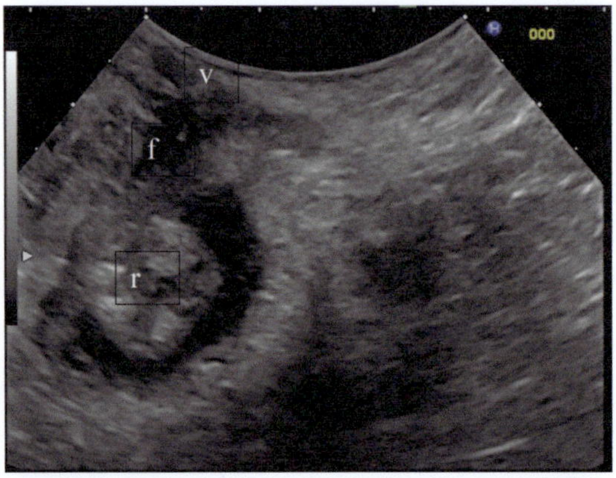

Fig. 8.11 Rectovaginal fistula. V = vagina, R = rectum, F = fistula

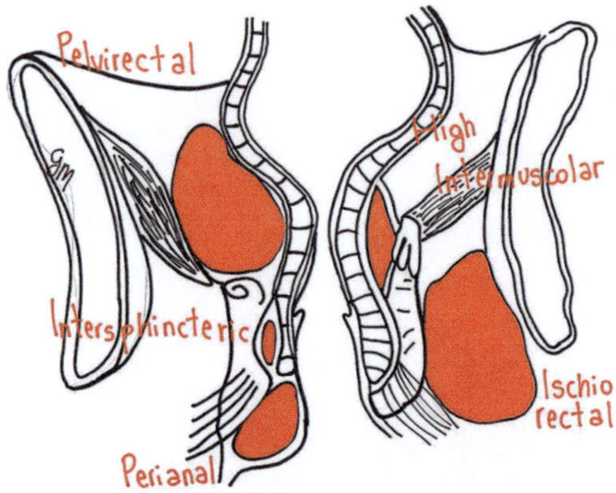

Fig. 8.13 Classification and site of perianal abscesses

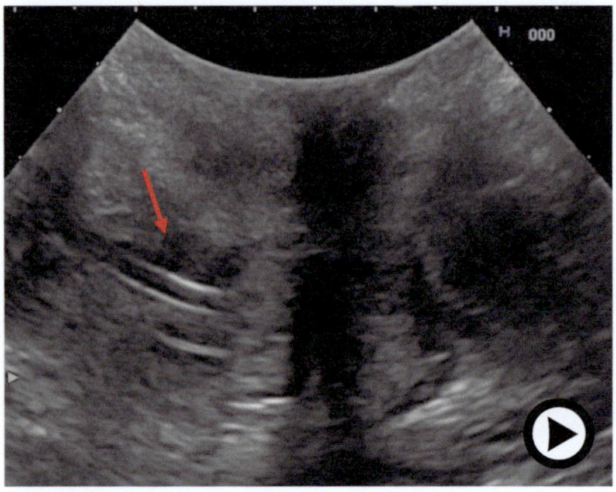

Fig. 8.12 Coronal scan. Seton is visible as two thin parallel hyperechoic bands (*arrow*) (▶ https://doi.org/10.1007/000-j2t)

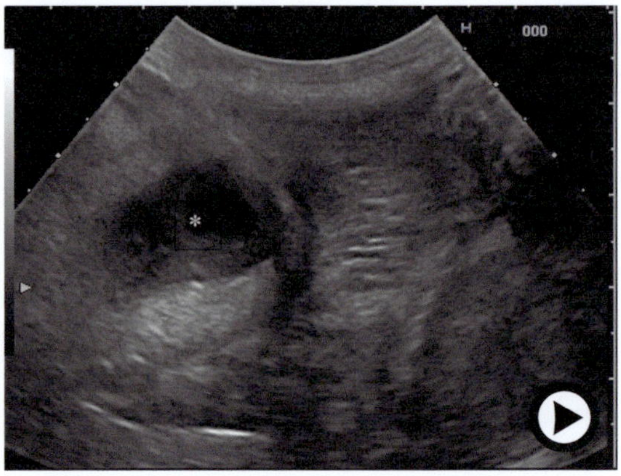

Fig. 8.14 Sagittal scan showing an ischioanal abscess (*) at the level of anorectal (▶ https://doi.org/10.1007/000-j2v)

TPUS can also identify perianal abscesses. Depending on their location, they are typically classified as pelvirectal, intersphincteric, ischiorectal, and superficial perianal abscesses (Fig. 8.13). The abscesses appear as hypoechoic or anechoic areas sometimes with inhomogeneous or gaseous content, with indistinct margins. The efficacy of TPUS in detecting deep pelvirectal abscesses, located superior to the levator ani muscle, may be limited. Intersphinteric abscess develops along the space between the internal and external sphincters, ischiorectal beyond the external sphincter (Fig. 8.14, Video 8.14), and perianal is located near the external anal orifice [7].

The evaluation of perianal lesions via TPUS can be significantly enhanced through the use of color Doppler (Fig. 8.15) and contrast-enhanced ultrasound (CEUS). Color Doppler and CEUS are particularly effective in visualizing the vascular characteristics of fistulas, potentially indicating their level of inflammatory activity.

Contrast-enhanced ultrasound (CEUS) is useful for identifying abscesses and small fluid collections within perianal inflammatory masses and fistulas. The abscess appears avascular in all phases of the study, whereas the phlegmon is vascularized.

Several studies have demonstrated that TPUS is an effective preliminary diagnostic tool for patients with suspected perianal fistulas and abscesses [8] or during follow-up in patients with

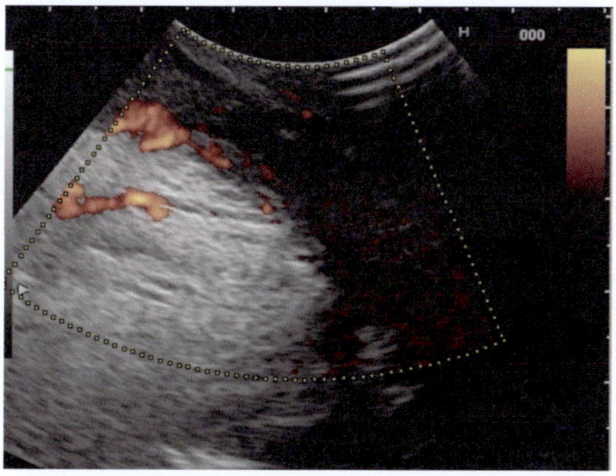

Fig. 8.15 Increased vascularization at the fistula walls on color Doppler

perianal fistulizing Crohn's disease under anti-TNF alpha therapy. This method is particularly useful for monitoring therapeutic response and detecting potential infectious complications during treatment, such as perianal abscesses [9].

Furthermore, TPUS can play a critical role in guiding clinical decisions regarding interventional or surgical treatments.

References

1. Nuernberg D, Saftoiu A, Barreiros AP, et al. EFSUMB commendations for gastrointestinal ultrasound part 3: endorectal, endoanal and perineal ultrasound. Ultrasound Int Open. 2019;5:E34–51.
2. Merz E. Transducer hygiene – an underrated topic? Ultraschall Med. 2005;26:7–8.
3. Sainio P. Fistula-in-ano in a defined population. Incidence and epidemiological aspects. Ann Chir Gynaecol. 1984;73:219–2.
4. Maconi G, Greco MT, Asthana AK. Transperineal ultrasound for perianal fistulas and abscesses—a systematic review and meta-analysis. Ultraschall Med. 2017;38:265–72.
5. Parks AG, Gordon PH, Hardcastle JD. A classification of fistula-in-ano. Br J Surg. 1976;63:1–12.
6. American Gastroenterological Association Clinical Practice Committee. American Gastroenterological Association medical position statement: perianal Crohn's disease. Gastroenterology. 2003;125:1503–7.
7. Lavazza A, Maconi G. Transperineal ultrasound for assessment of fistulas and abscesses: a pictorial essay. J Ultrasound. 2019;22(2):241–9.
8. Terracciano F, Scalisi G, Bossa F, et al. Transperineal ultrasonography: first level exam in IBD patients with perianal disease. Dig Liver Dis. 2016;48:874–9.
9. Rasul I, Wlson SR, MacRae H, et al. Clinical and radiological response after infliximab treatment for perianal fistulizing Crohn's disease. Am J Gastroenterol. 2003;99:82–8.

9 Intestinal Ultrasound in Pediatric Inflammatory Bowel

Ramit Magen-Rimon

9.1 Introduction

The incidence of pediatric inflammatory bowel diseases (IBD) is steadily increasing and the diagnosis age is declining worldwide [1–3].

Strict monitoring of disease activity is important and can prevent pubertal delay and failure to thrive. It is also important to assess disease complications, such as fistula formation, intra-abdominal abscesses, and intestinal strictures as well as pre-stenotic dilatation.

Noninvasive methods for monitoring disease activity pose challenges in the pediatric population. Computed tomography (CT) exposes patients to radiation, especially concerning long-term follow-up. Magnetic resonance enterography (MRE) requires a patient's cooperation, often difficult in pediatric patients, particularly younger ones.

Consequently, intestinal ultrasound (IUS) emerges as the preferred noninvasive tool for assessing disease activity, location, and complications in this population. IUS is favored due to its bedside feasibility, cost-effectiveness, and lack of radiation exposure.

Intestinal ultrasound (IUS) demonstrates a sensitivity of 70% and specificity of 96% in diagnosing bowel inflammation in pediatric patients [4]. Several studies in both adults and children have shown IUS to be comparable to MRE in evaluating disease activity and complications [5, 6].

Despite its advantages, IUS has limitations, notably the challenge of visualizing the rectum. However, this can sometimes be overcome by using a convex probe positioned above the pubic bone directed towards the rectum (Fig. 9.1).

Supplementary Information: The online version contains supplementary material available at https://doi.org/10.1007/978-3-032-11418-1_9. The videos can be accessed individually by clicking the DOI link in the accompanying figure caption or by scanning this link with the SN More Media App.

R. Magen-Rimon (✉)
Pediatric Gastroenterology & Nutrition Institute, Ruth Children's Hospital of Haifa, Rambam Medical Center, Haifa, Israel

Faculty of Medicine, Technion, Haifa, Israel

F. Terracciano et al. (eds.), *Bowel Ultrasound Compared with Endoscopy*, https://doi.org/10.1007/978-3-032-11418-1_9

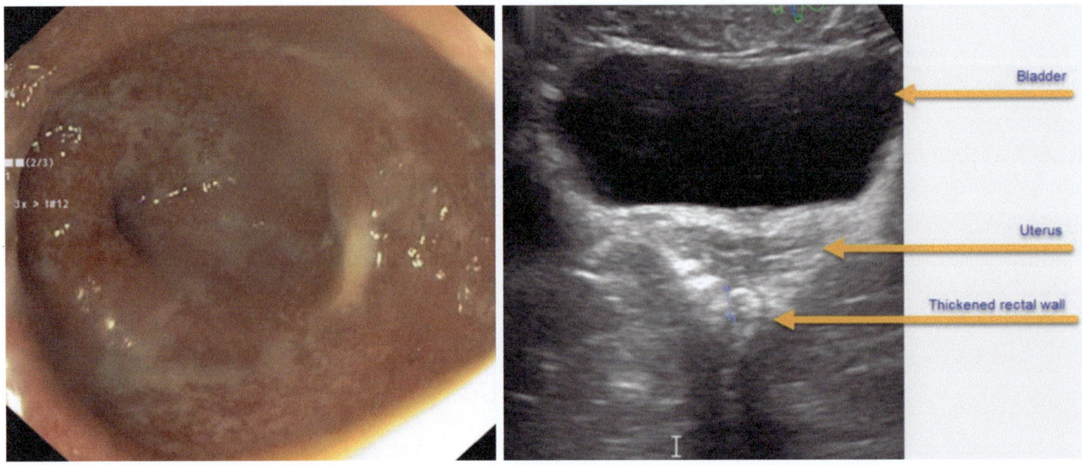

Fig. 9.1 Colonoscopy demonstrating inflamed rectum with hyperemic and edematous mucosa and exudates. On the right is the sonographic image of the rectum visualized using a convex probe positioned proximal to the pubic bone

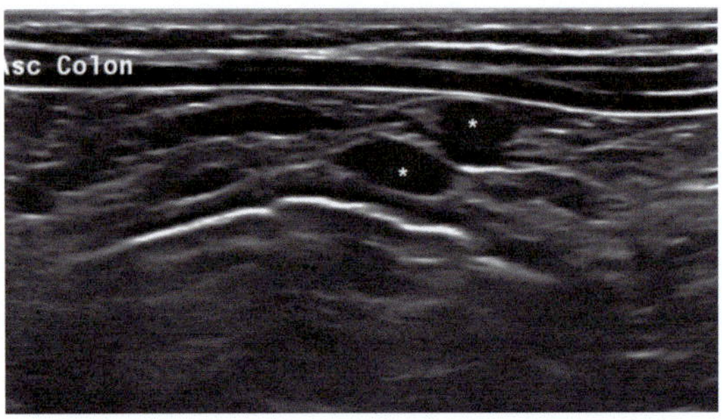

Fig. 9.2 Lymph node enlargement can be identified as oval or round hypoecoic structures and can be distinguished from blood vesseles by utilization of color Doppler imaging (*asterisks*)

9.2 Disease Activity Indices

Indices of disease activity in IBD are primarily characterized by bowel wall thickening, increased color Doppler signaling (indicating hyperemia) that reflects hyperemia, and loss of bowel wall layers. Additional indicators include lymph nodes enlargement (Fig. 9.2) and hyperechoic inflamed mesenteric fat (Fig. 9.3).

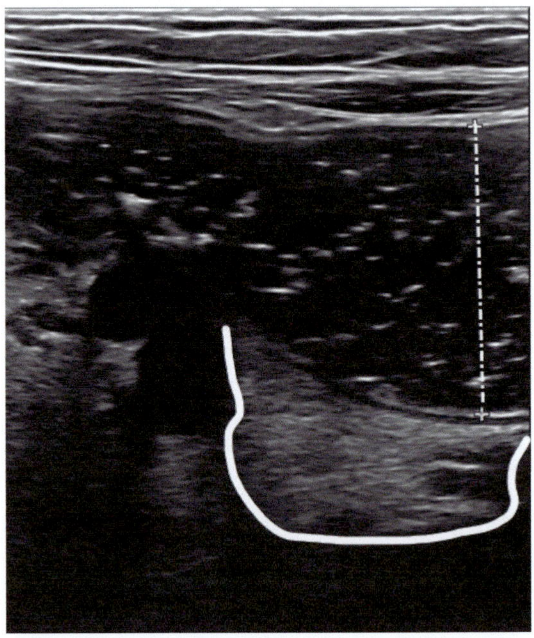

Fig. 9.3 Pre-stenotic dilatation (*dashed line*) and inflamed, hyperechoic mesenteric fat (*full line*)

9.2.1 Bowel Wall Thickening

In an adequate image of the intestinal wall, it is possible to discern five distinct layers. The inner layer, visualized as a hyperechoic layer, represents the interface between the lumen and mucosa. Moving outward, one can observe the hypoechoic mucosal layer, followed by the hyperechoic submucosa, the hypoechoic muscularis propria, and finally, the hyperechoic serosa (Figs. 9.4 and 9.5).

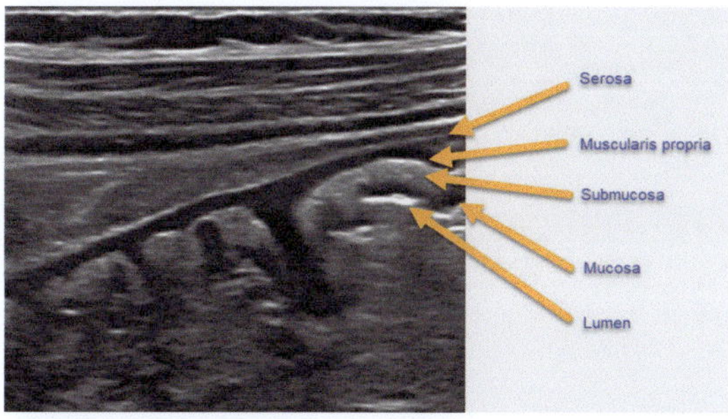

Fig. 9.4 Thickened submucosa in an inflamed colon segment with preserved haustra

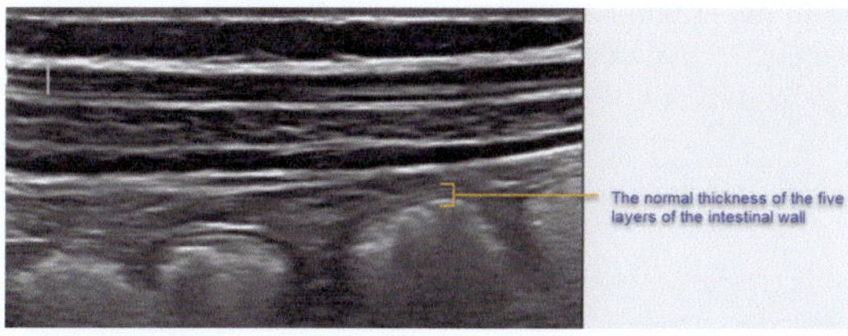

Fig. 9.5 Normal segment of the colon from the same patient exhibits preserved haustra and normal bowel wall thickness (Limberg score 0)

It is important to note that intestinal bowel thickening can result from fibrosis in long-standing disease, and is not specific to intestinal inflammation [7]. Thus, other signs of inflammation should be considered.

Miyoshi et al. [8] demonstrated that a thickened submucosa predicts an inflammatory process in ulcerative colitis (UC), even when total bowel wall thickness is normal (<2 mm). This observation was supported by a study correlating sonographic features with histologic evaluation of resected small bowel specimen. This study [9] also demonstrated a correlation between thickened mucosal layer and intestinal fibrosis, although both mucosal and submucosal thickening are features of intestinal active inflammation.

The normal upper limit of for intestinal bowel thickness in children is inconsistently reported, ranging between 1.5–3 mm in the terminal ileum (TI) and 2 mm for colon [7, 10]. A meta-analysis of 7 studies comprising of 207 healthy children under 18, found the upper limit of normal bowel thickness to be 1.9 mm for both small and large intestines with up to 0.5 mm increase in adolescents between 15 and 18 years compared to younger children (<4 years old), showing thicker jejunal and colonic wall in the older children [11].

Van Wassenaer and colleagues [10] found that in the pediatric population, a colonic wall thickness exceeding 2 mm combined with mesenteric fat inflammation or a threshold of >3.7 and >2.7 in TI and colon, respectively, in the absence of any other mentioned sonographic indicators of inflammation, serves as a predictive marker for endoscopically active disease.

In pediatric patients with IBD, emerging data suggests a cutoff of 3 mm for small bowel and <2 mm for colon [12].

9.2.2 Color Doppler Imaging

Hyperemia of the bowel is expressed by Limberg score [13]. This score, while semi-quantitative, is subjective, and therefore depends on the evaluator's judgment.

Limberg 0—Normal bowel wall thickness and no color Doppler signal (Fig. 9.5)

Limberg 1—Increased bowel wall thickness with no color Doppler signal (Fig. 9.6)

Limberg 2—Increased bowel wall thickness with intermittent signaling, presented as spots within the bowel wall (Video 9.1; Fig. 9.7)

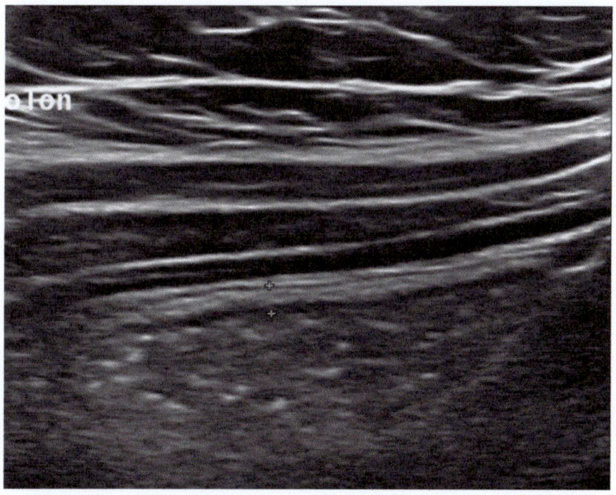

Fig. 9.6 Limberg score 1—thickened bowel wall with no vascularization (*calipers*)

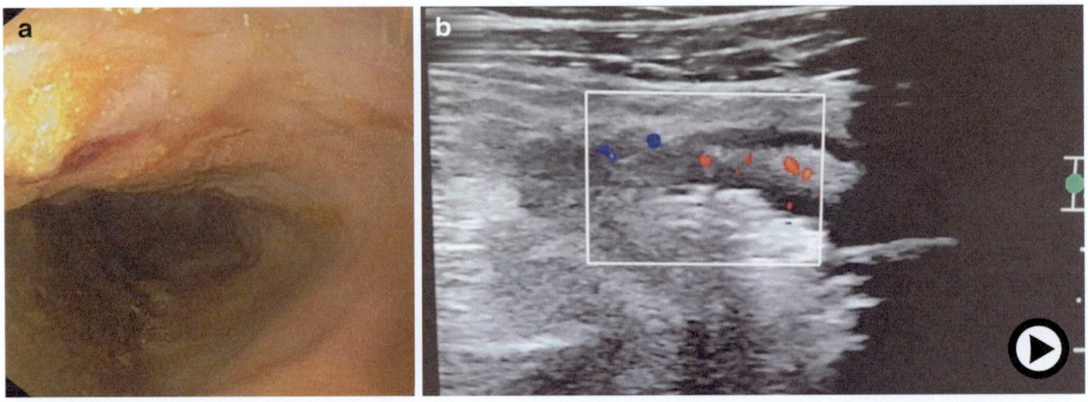

Fig. 9.7 Sixteen-year-old patient with Crohn's disease. (**a**) Colonoscopy demonstrating edematous terminal ileum and few aphthae. (**b**) On the right—IUS demonstrating terminal ileitis with thickened bowel wall and mild hyperemia—Limberg score 2 (Video 9.1 Mild intermittent hyperemia and thickened bowel wall (▶ https://doi.org/10.1007/000-j2y))

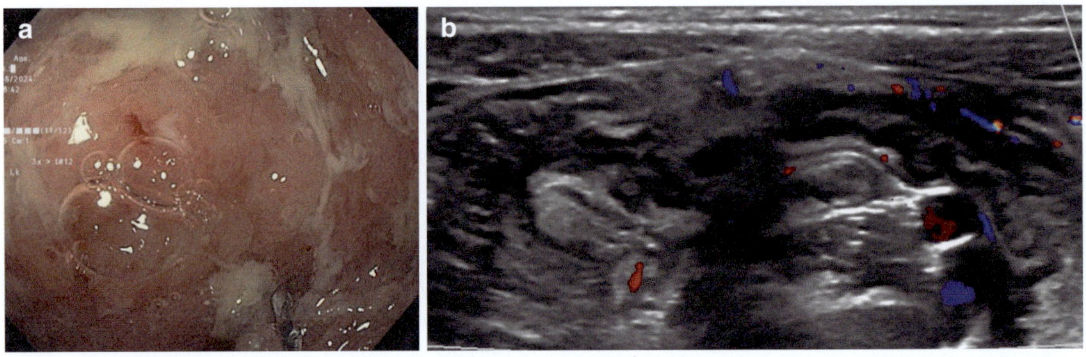

Fig. 9.8 Nine years old female with terminal ileitis. (**a**) Colonoscopy demonstrating terminal ileitis with ulcerations. (**b**) The corresponding IUS image thickened TI and hyperemia with Limberg score 3 with protracted stretches of vascularity

Limberg 3—Increased bowel wall thickness with protracted stretches of increased vascularity through the bowel wall (Fig. 9.8)

Limberg 4—Increased bowel wall thickness with color Doppler signals extend beyond the bowel wall to the surrounding mesenteric fat (Fig. 9.9c, d; Video 9.2)

9.2.3 Loss of Bowel Wall Layers Stratification

This characteristics corresponds to deep ulcers and severe inflammation [7] (Fig. 9.9c, d).

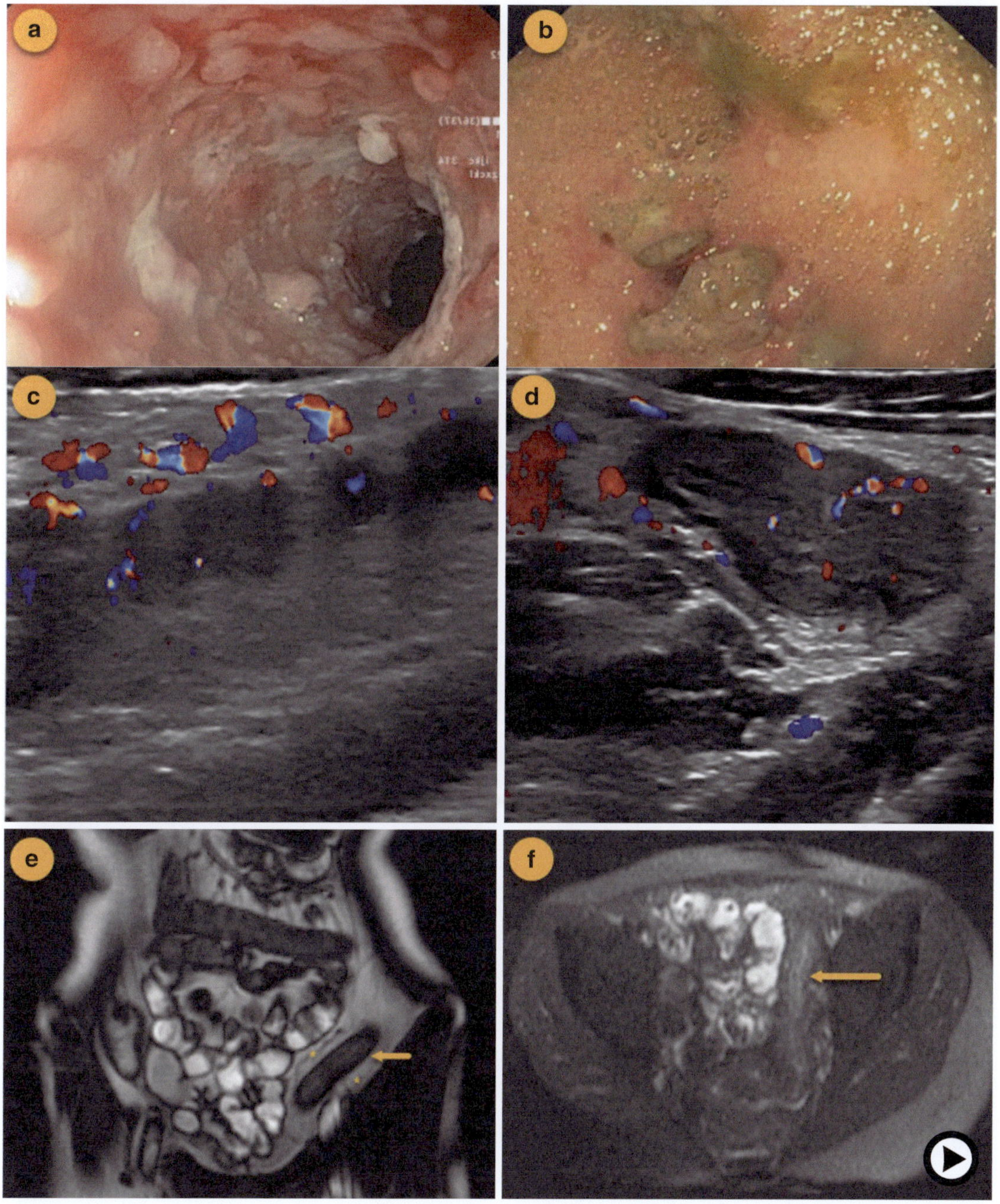

Fig. 9.9 Crohn's colitis in a 12-year-old female. (**a**, **b**) Colonoscopy demonstrating deep ulcers, exudates, and friable tissue as well as pseudo polyps. (**c**, **d**) Sonographic image demonstrating loss of bowel wall layers stratification and severe hyperemia—Limberg score 4 (Video 9.2 Limberg score 4, fistula (▶ https://doi.org/10.1007/000-j2x)). (**e**, **f**) MRE coronal and axial view demonstrating thickened colonic wall (arrows) and hypertrophied mesenteric fat (stars)

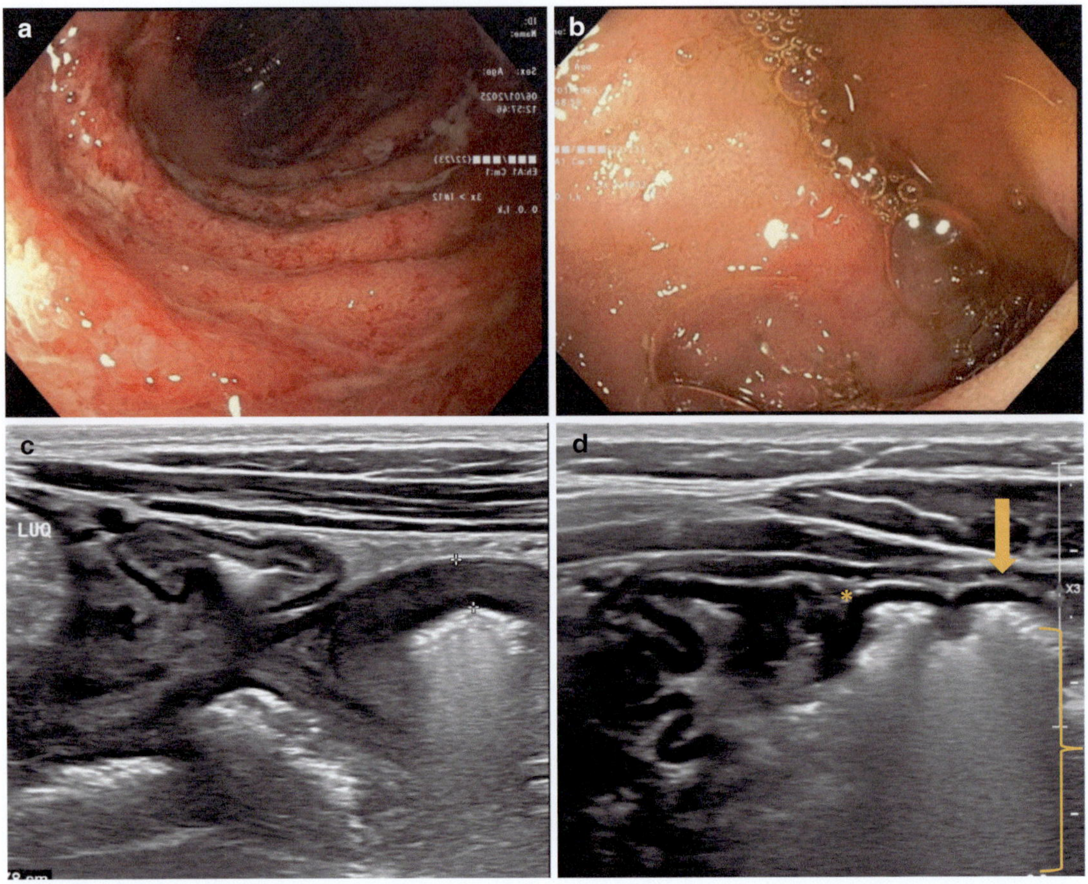

Fig. 9.10 Eleven-year-old female with stricturing Crohn's disease, primarily affecting the small intestine. (**a**) Enteroscopy demonstrating inflamed Jejunum. (**b**) Pre-stenotic duodenal dilatation without inflammation. (**c**) Sonographic image of the same patient. Thickened jejunal submucosa prior to treatment (*calipers*). (**d**) The same patient 2 months after treatment initiation—less thickened submucosa (*asterisks*) with pre-stenotic dilatation (*arrow*)

9.3 Crohn's Disease Imaging

9.3.1 Strictures and Pre-stenotic Dilatation

Pediatric patients more frequently present with extensive disease and upper GI involvement as compared to adults [14]. The jejunum is located in the left upper quadrant and is characterized by a distinct folds pattern (Fig. 9.10). Small bowel luminal diameter may fluctuate due to peristalsis following recent food ingestion; however, in adults, a diameter exceeding 3 cm is considered abnormal and corresponds to pre-stenotic dilata-

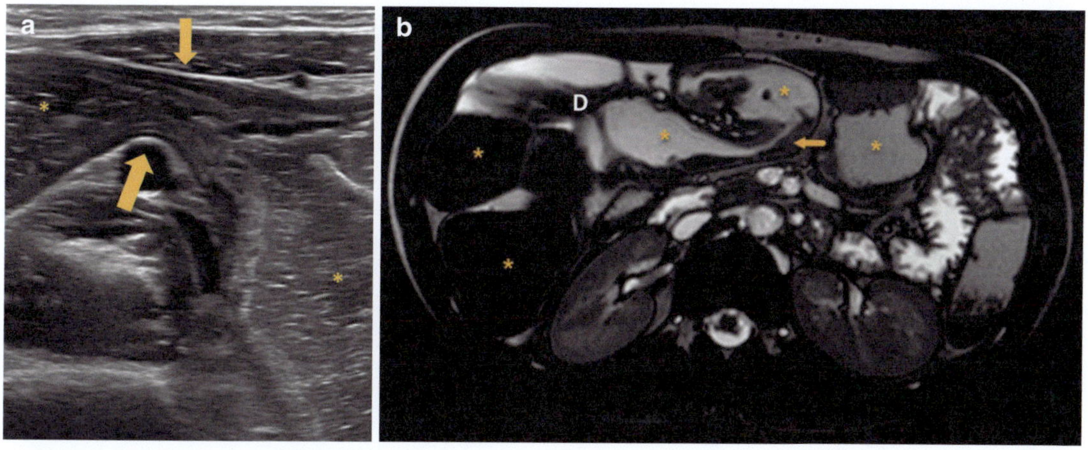

Fig. 9.11 Fifteen-year-old male with stricturing Crohn's disease, primarily affecting the small intestine. (**a**) Sonographic imaging demonstrates small bowel stricture (*arrows*), pre- and post-stenotic dilatation (*asterisks*). (**b**) MRE image of the same patient demonstrating several dilated small bowel loops (*asterisks*) and stricture (*arrow*) with intestinal wall thickening and narrowed lumen. Normal small intestine can be observed on the right side

tion whereas a luminal narrowing less than 1 cm suggests a stricture (Fig. 9.11) [15].

9.3.2 Fistulae and Abscesses

Areas of tethered mesentery and intestinal loops or loops adjacent to other organs or bowel loops are suggestive of fistula formation.

Fistulas appear as hypoechoic tracts that project from an inflamed bowel wall to another adjacent organ (bladder, intestinal loop, colon, mesentery, psoas muscle) [7] (Video 9.3; Fig. 9.12).

Abscesses can be recognized as hypoechoic masses without well-defined borders (Figs. 9.12 and 9.13).

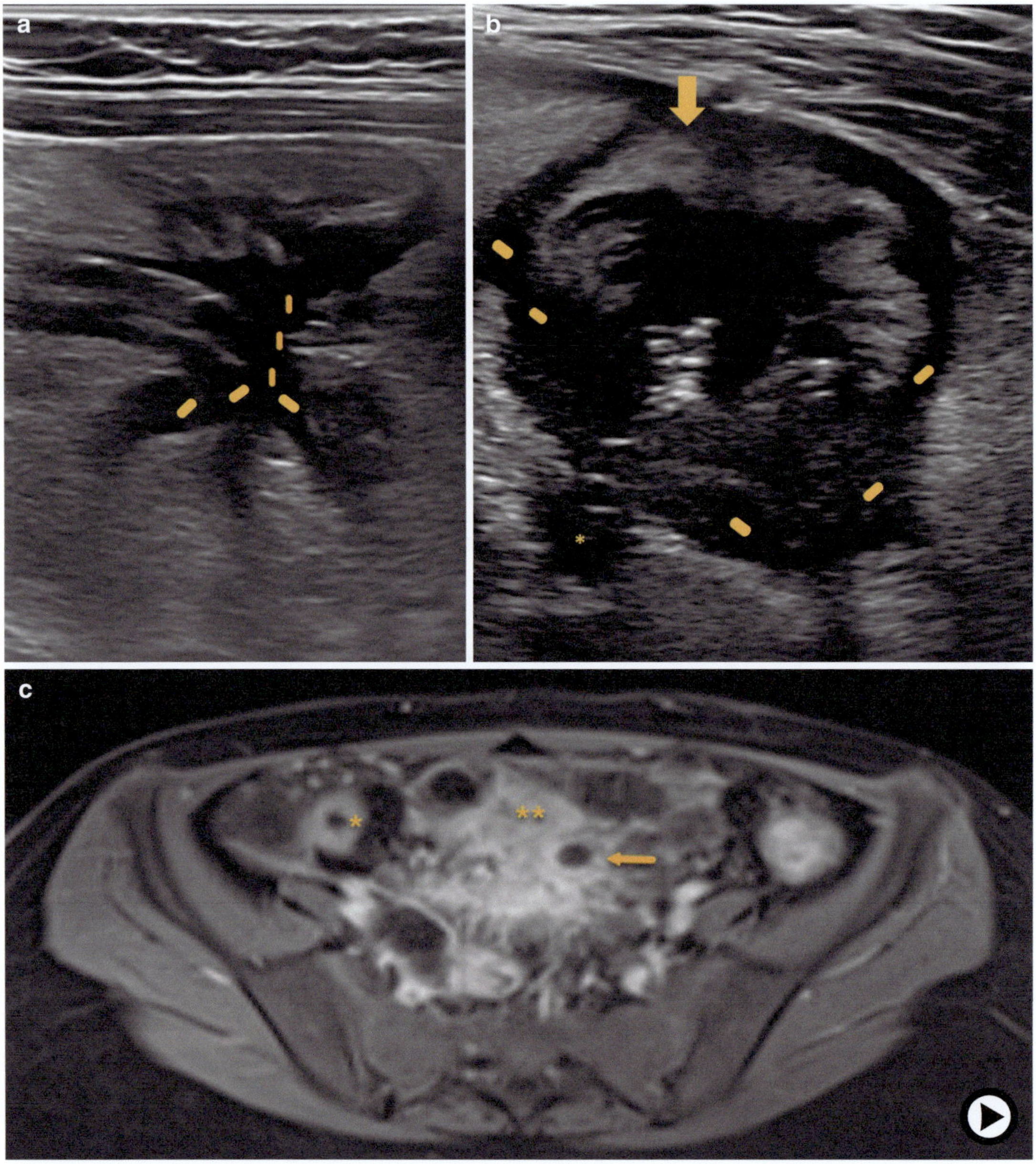

Fig. 9.12 Penetrating CD. (**a**) An ultrasound image demonstrating fistula tracts connecting two adjacent segments of small intestine and extending into the mesentery (*dashed line*) (Video 9.3 Fistula and inflamed mesentery (▶ https://doi.org/10.1007/000-j2w)). (**b**) Thickened small bowel wall with loss of stratification (*arrow*), fistulas (*dashed lines*), and a small abscess. (**c**) An axial view of MRE demonstrating inflamed intestine with a thickened wall (*asterisk*), a tethered mesentery (*double asterisks*), and an abscess (*arrow*)

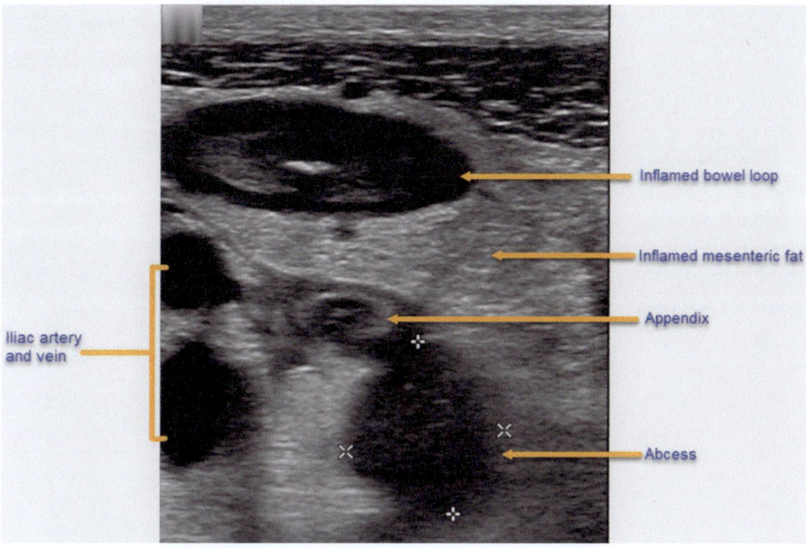

Fig. 9.13 Fifteen-year-old patient with Crohn's disease presenting with peri-appendicular abscess (*calipers*) and adjacent inflamed intestine with thickened bowel wall, loss of wall layers stratification, and inflamed surrounding mesenteric fat

9.4 Ulcerative Colitis Imaging

In the pediatric population, as opposed to the adult UC patients, colonic involvement is typically extensive and most frequently present as pancolitis [14]. The sonographic features of inflammation intensify progressively as the scan advances toward the distal colon (Video 9.4).

The endoscopic Mayo scores and the corresponding IUS images are presented in Fig. 9.14a–g.

The colon's lead pipe appearance is observed in chronic colitis [16] (Fig. 9.15; Video 9.4). This appearance results from the contraction of the hypertrophied muscularis mucosa, which leads to the loss of haustra [16].

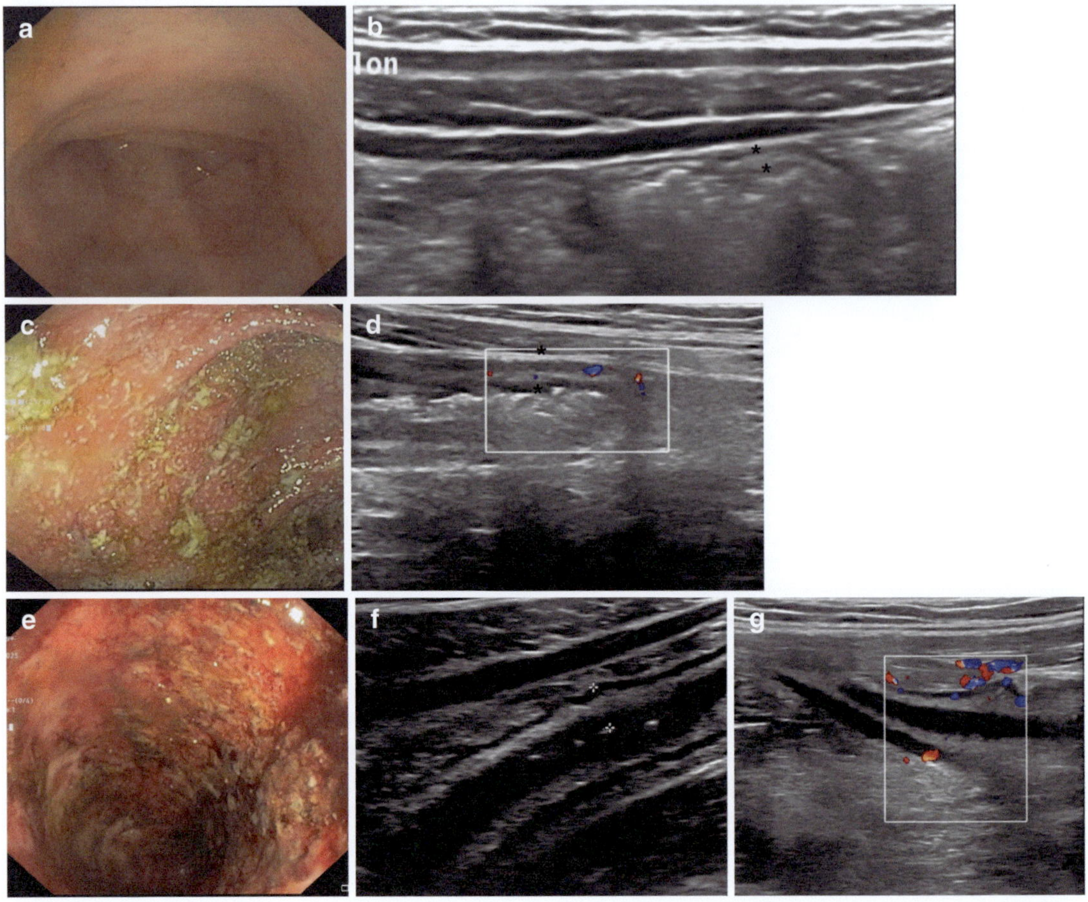

Fig. 9.14 (**a**) Mayo endoscopic score 1—edema and mild erythema. (**b**) The corresponding IUS image demonstrating mild thickening of the bowel wall, with predominantly thickening of the sub-mucosa layer (*asterisks*). (**c**) Mayo endoscopic score 2—marked erythema, edema, and erosions. (**d**) Increased bowel wall thickening (*asterisks*) with hyperemia (Limberg score 2). (**e**) Mayo score 3—ulcerations and spontaneous bleeding. (**f**, **g**) Markedly increased bowel wall thickening (*calipers*), loss of stratification, Limberg score 4

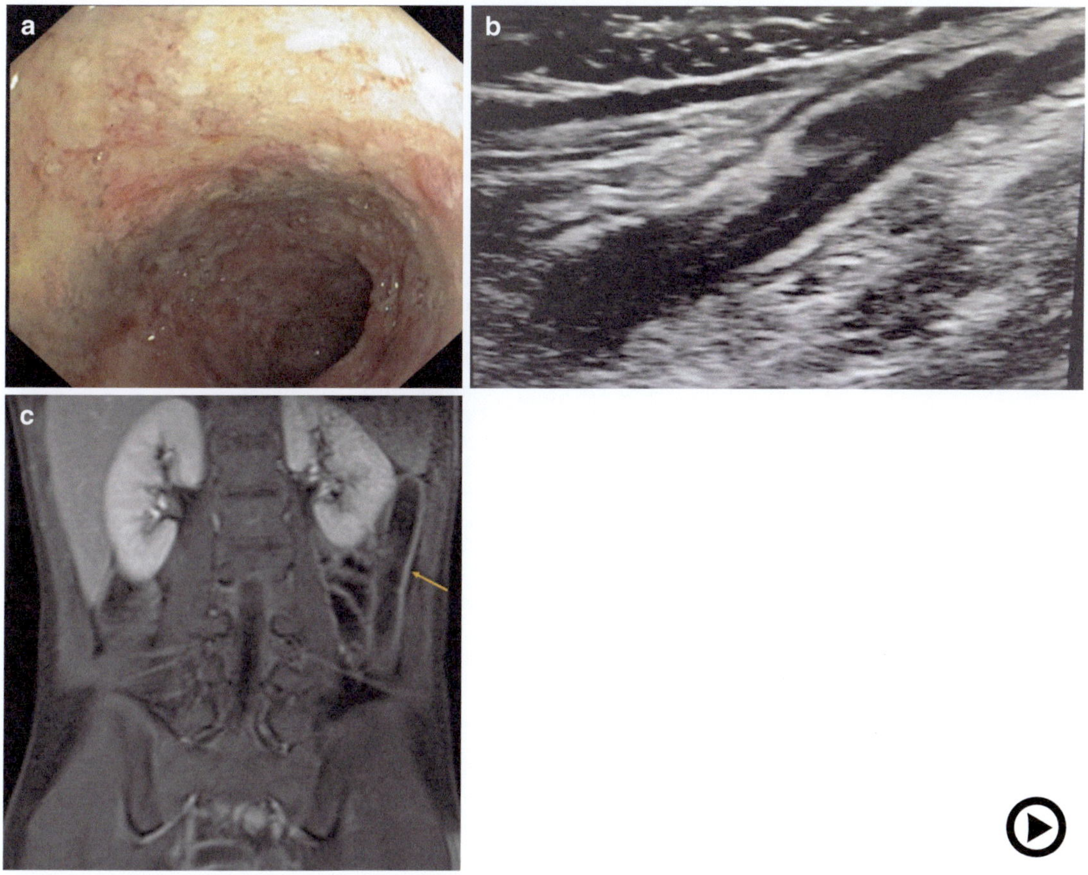

Fig. 9.15 Patient with ulcerative colitis. (**a**) Colonoscopy demonstrates pancolitis with fibrin, erythema, as well as lead pipe appearance (Mayo endoscopic score 3). (**b**) Intestinal ultrasound demonstrating pancolitis with lead pipe appearance due to the loss of haustra (Video 9.4 Pancolitis, lead pipe appearance, bowel wall thickening (▶ https://doi.org/10.1007/000-j2z)). (**c**) MRE coronal view demonstrating lead pipe appearance of the colon (*arrow*)

References

1. Benchimol EI, Bernstein CN, Bitton A, Carroll MW, Singh H, Otley AR, et al. Trends in epidemiology of pediatric inflammatory bowel disease in Canada: distributed network analysis of multiple population-based provincial health administrative databases. Am J Gastroenterol. 2017;112(7):1120–34.
2. Sýkora J, Pomahačová R, Kreslová M, Cvalínová D, Štych P, Schwarz J. Current global trends in the incidence of pediatric-onset inflammatory bowel disease. World J Gastroenterol. 2018;24:2741–63.
3. Choe JY, Choi S, Song KH, Jang HJ, Choi KH, Yi DY, et al. Incidence and prevalence trends of pediatric inflammatory bowel disease in the Daegu-Kyungpook Province from 2017 to 2020. Front Pediatr. 2022;9(January):1–7.
4. Dilillo D, Zuccotti GV, Galli E, Meneghin F, Dell'Era A, Penagini F, et al. Noninvasive testing in the management of children with suspected inflammatory bowel disease. Scand J Gastroenterol. 2019;54(5):586–91.
5. Allocca M, Fiorino G, Bonifacio C, Furfaro F, Gilardi D, Argollo M, et al. Comparative accuracy of bowel ultrasound versus magnetic resonance enterography in combination with colonoscopy in assessing Crohn's disease and guiding clinical decision-making. J Crohns Colitis. 2018;12(11):1280–7.
6. Dillman JR, Smith EA, Sanchez RJ, DiPietro MA, DeMatos-Maillard V, Strouse PJ, et al. Pediatric small bowel Crohn disease: correlation of US and MR enterography. Radiographics. 2015;35(3):835–48.
7. Alison M, Kheniche A, Azoulay R, Roche S, Sebag G, Belarbi N. Ultrasonography of Crohn disease in children. Pediatr Radiol. 2007;37(11):1071–82.

8. Miyoshi J, Ozaki R, Yonezawa H, Mori H, Kawamura N, Matsuura M, et al. Ratio of submucosal thickness to total bowel wall thickness as a new sonographic parameter to estimate endoscopic remission of ulcerative colitis. J Gastroenterol [Internet]. 2022;57(2):82–9. Available from: https://doi.org/10.1007/s00535-021-01847-3.
9. Bhatnagar G, Rodriguez-Justo M, Higginson A, Bassett P, Windsor A, Cohen R, et al. Inflammation and fibrosis in Crohn's disease: location-matched histological correlation of small bowel ultrasound features. Abdom Radiol [Internet]. 2021;46(1):144–55. Available from: https://doi.org/10.1007/s00261-020-02603-6.
10. van Wassenaer EA, van Rijn RR, de Voogd FAE, van Schuppen J, Kindermann A, de Meij TGJ, et al. Assessing disease activity in pediatric Crohn's disease using ultrasound: the pediatric Crohn disease intestinal ultrasound score. J Pediatr Gastroenterol Nutr. 2023;76(5):582–9.
11. Van Wassenaer EA, De Voogd FAE, Van Rijn RR, Van Der Lee JH, Tabbers MM, Van Etten-Jamaludin FS, et al. Diagnostic accuracy of transabdominal ultrasound in detecting intestinal inflammation in paediatric IBD patients – a systematic review. J Crohns Colitis. 2019;13(12):1501–9.
12. Kellar A, Dolinger M, Novak KL, Chavannes M, Dubinsky M, Huynh H. Intestinal ultrasound for the pediatric gastroenterologist: a guide for inflammatory bowel disease monitoring in children: expert consensus on behalf of the International Bowel Ultrasound Group (IBUS) Pediatric Committee. J Pediatr Gastroenterol Nutr. 2023;76(2):142–8.
13. Limberg B. Diagnosis of chronic inflammatory bowel disease by ultrasonography. Z Gastroenterol. 1999;37(6):495–508.
14. Kahn SA. The transition from pediatric to adult inflammatory bowel disease care. Gastroenterol Hepatol. 2016;12(6):403–6.
15. Rieder F, Bettenworth D, Ma C, Parker CE, Lee A, Nelson SA, et al. An expert consensus to standardize definitions, diagnosis and treatment targets for antifibrotic stricture therapies in Crohn's disease. Aliment Pharmacol Ther. 2019;48(3):347–57.
16. Baldwin M, Genant J, Braver J, Mortele KJ. Classic signs in gastrointestinal radiology. Appl Radiol. 2012;41(4):35A.

Other Ultrasonographic Intestinal Findings in Pediatric Patients

10

Francesco Esposito, Dolores Ferrara, Anna Masucci, and Francesca Antonia De Chiara

10.1 Pediatric Ultrasound Anatomy

The gastrointestinal ultrasound anatomy in pediatrics is essentially similar to that of adults. The main structures of the gastrointestinal tract are visualized in similar ways, including the organ walls and their distinct ultrasound layers [1]. However, certain specific differences exist in the pediatric context [2]. Specifically, ultrasound examination of the subdiaphragmatic portion of the esophagus (Fig. 10.1) requires particular adjustments in children, due to its position and relative size. Using high-frequency probes and optimal angling enhance visibility in this region. Another significant difference involves the terminal ileal loops, where the lymphoid component is more pronounced in children. Peyer's patches, lymphoid structures located in the ileal mucosa, are more prominent compared to adults, plaing a crucial role in immune response, and are well-visualized on ultrasound as hypoechoic thickenings (Fig. 10.2). This lymphoid aspect is especially evident in the presence of intestinal inflammation or infection [1].

F. Esposito (✉) · D. Ferrara
Emergency Radiology Department, Santobono-Pausilipon Children Hospital, Naples, Italy
e-mail: f.esposito2@santobonopausilipon.it

A. Masucci
Department of Radiology, University "Federico II", Naples, Italy

F. A. De Chiara
Department of Radiology, University of Molise, Campobasso, Italy

F. Terracciano et al. (eds.), *Bowel Ultrasound Compared with Endoscopy*,
https://doi.org/10.1007/978-3-032-11418-1_10

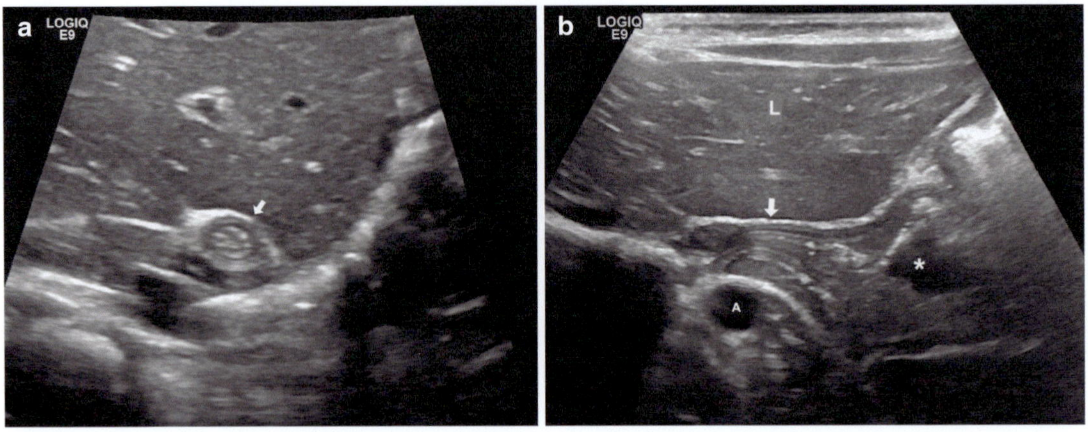

Fig. 10.1 Subdiaphragmatic esophagus. (**a**) In axial scan, the esophagus appears as a "target" image (arrow). (**b**) In longitudinal scan the esophagus appears as a tubular structure (arrow) visualized behind the liver (L). (A) abdominal aorta; (*) lumen of the stomach

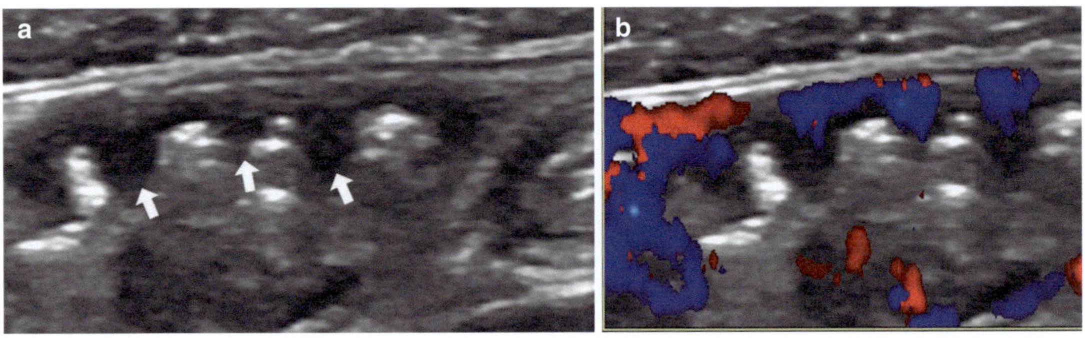

Fig. 10.2 Ileal terminal loop. (**a**) The image shows hypertrophy of the mucosal folds (arrows). (**b**) Color Doppler demonstrates the presence of increased vascularization of the mucosa

10.2 Hypertrophic Pyloric Stenosis

Hypertrophic pyloric stenosis (HPS) is a condition that typically arises between 2 and 8 weeks of life, manifesting with characteristic "projectile" vomiting that occurs immediately after feeding [1]. This non-bilious vomiting becomes progressively more frequent and forceful, posing risks of dehydration and growth arrest if not promptly treated. Clinical suspicion is mainly based on symptoms and the possible presence of a small, round palpable mass in the epigastric area, commonly referred to as an "olive" due to its shape [1, 3]. HPS is characterized by abnormal thickening of the circular muscle of the pyloric sphincter, which becomes four times thicker than the surrounding longitudinal musculature. This thickening of the pylorus causes a significant narrowing of the pyloric canal, making food passage from the stomach to the intestine difficult. As the condition progresses, the canal tends to lengthen further, and the mucosa thickens, exacerbating the problem of gastric emptying. Ultrasound is now the primary tool for diagnosing HPS and is extremely accurate in visualizing the pyloric region [1, 3, 4]. During the ultrasound examination, performed with the infant in the supine position, a high-frequency linear probe (7.5–14 MHz) is used, focusing on the sub-xiphoid and right paramedian region. For optimal visualization of the pylorus, the stomach

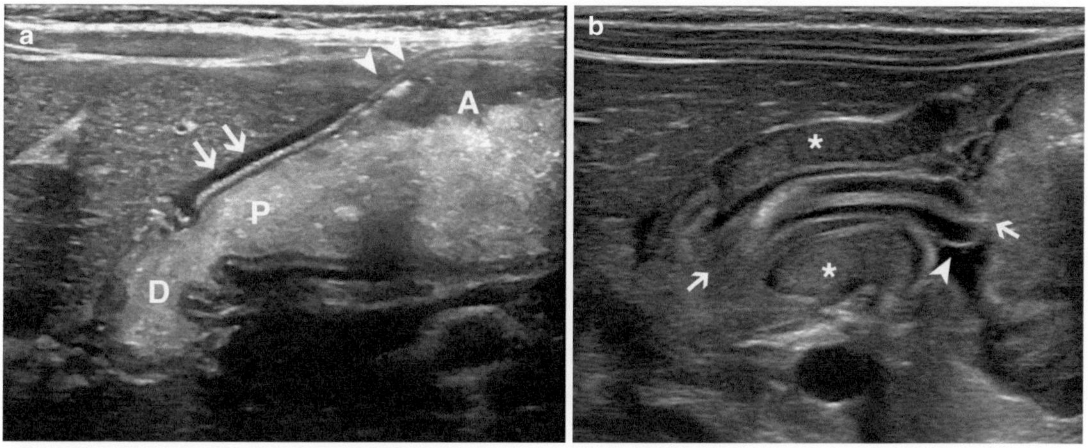

Fig. 10.3 Pyloric stenosis. Long-axis scan. (**a**) The image shows the appearance of a normal pylorus. The walls of the pylorus (arrows) show the same thickness and layering as found in the walls of the gastric antrum (arrowheads). (**b**) The image shows thickening of the muscular layer (*) and elongation of the pyloric canal (arrows). "Cervix sign" determined by the protrusion of the mucosa into the gastric antrum (arrowhead) is also visible. P pylorus, D duodenum, A gastric antrum

should not be completely empty, as excessive gastric distension could complicate visualization due to posterior displacement of the pylorus. The normal pylorus shows walls similar in thickness to those of the gastric antrum; moreover, the wall layers show the same thickness (Fig. 10.3a).

In HPS the typical ultrasound appearance of the thickened pylorus can be visualized in two views: in an axial scan, the pylorus appears as a "target," and in a longitudinal scan, it appears as an elongated and often curved structure (Fig. 10.3b). The thickened pyloric muscle appears hypoechoic (darker than surrounding tissues) and may sometimes present irregular echogenicity due to anisotropy issues, especially during muscle contraction, giving the pylorus a "striped" appearance. Ultrasound diagnostic criteria for HPS include a pyloric canal length exceeding 18 mm and a muscular thickness of 4 mm or more [1, 3, 4]. However, in premature or low birth-weight infants, these parameters may vary, and slightly lower values could still indicate the condition. Other important accessory signs include curvature of the pyloric canal, pyloric protrusion into the duodenum (the "portio" sign), and the "railroad" appearance of the thickened pyloric mucosa protruding into the gastric antrum (known as the "cervix" or "nipple sign") [3]. In cases of diagnostic uncertainty, especially with borderline muscle thickness, follow-up ultrasound examination 1–2 weeks apart can be helpful. Dynamic ultrasound assessment also allows for the evaluation of gastric antrum contractility and the degree of pyloric canal opening. In infants with HPS, the pyloric canal remains closed or insufficiently distended, and the muscle remains thickened. Another common sign is gastric distension, often accompanied by gastroesophageal reflux. In summary, ultrasound provides a detailed and precise picture of HPS, allowing visualization of the muscle thickening and narrowing of the pyloric canal, confirming the diagnosis with high reliability through clear parameters such as pyloric length and thickness.

10.3 Intussusception

Intestinal intussusception is a common cause of intestinal obstruction in children, especially between 4 and 8 months of age, with a higher prevalence in males [1, 5]. It is a condition in which a portion of the intestine (intussusceptum) pushes into an adjacent distal part (intussuscipiens), causing vascular compression and potentially leading to ischemia, edema, and bleeding, manifested by symptoms like bloody, mucus-containing stools ("red currant jelly" stool). Ultrasound is the diagnostic tool of choice for intestinal intussusception, with near 100% sensitivity and accuracy [1, 5, 6]. Sonographically, intussusception appears, in short-axis view, as an intestinal mass, usually located in the right flank, with a diameter between 20 and 50 mm., with alternating concentric hyperechoic and hypoechoic rings ("target sign" or "doughnut sign") (Fig. 10.4). Ultrasound distinguishes various forms of intussusception:

1. Ileo-colic: the most common, often idiopathic
2. Ileo-ileal: generally benign and transient
3. Colo-colic: the rarest, often due to polyps or other structural anomalies

Ultrasound is useful not only for diagnosis but also for evaluating the success of hydrostatic or pneumatic reductions, which are essential for resolving intussusception without surgery [5].

10.4 Duplication Cyst

An enteric duplication cyst is a rare congenital anomaly that can develop anywhere along the digestive tract, from the mouth to the anus. Most commonly, it is found in the small intestine, especially the distal ileum, typically on the mesenteric side of the lumen [1, 7]. Duplication cysts may be cystic or tubular and contain fluid. Structurally, they consist of an inner lining of gastrointestinal epithelium and an outer layer of smooth muscle. The tubular variant, which is less common, is directly connected to the intestinal lumen, unlike the spherical form. The exact cause of duplication cysts is unknown, but the most accepted theory involves abnormal recanalization of the intestinal lumen during embryonic development. Clinical presentation varies depending on location, relative mass effect, and complications associated with the secretion of the involved epithelium. Patients with duplication cysts in the small intestine may present with symptoms such as vomiting and abdominal pain. Duodenal cysts may cause complications such as pancreatitis, infections, weight loss, and gastrointestinal bleeding due to ectopic gastric mucosa [1]. Jejunal cysts can cause

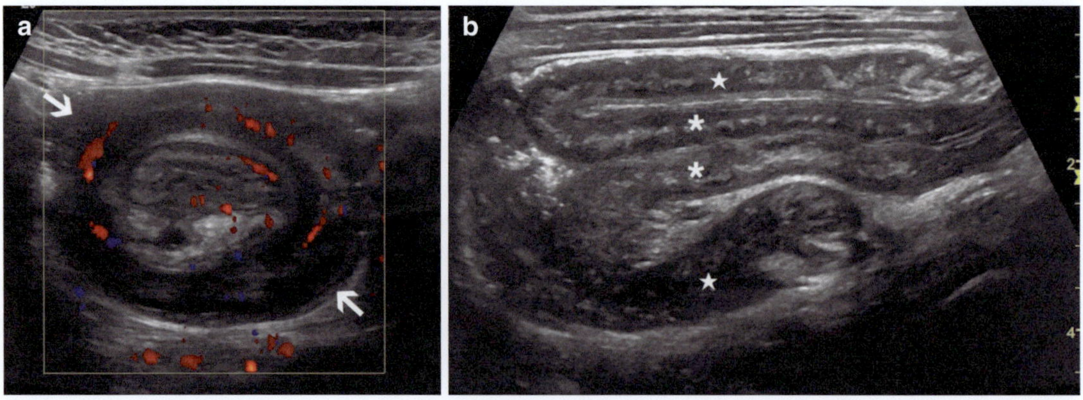

Fig. 10.4 Intussusception. (**a**) Short-axis scan shows a large structure (arrows) with concentric hypo echoic and hyperechoic rings ("Target" sign). (**b**) Long-axis scan shows the invagination of a proximal segment of intestine, the intussusceptum (*) into a more caudal segment of bowel, the intussuscipiens (stars)

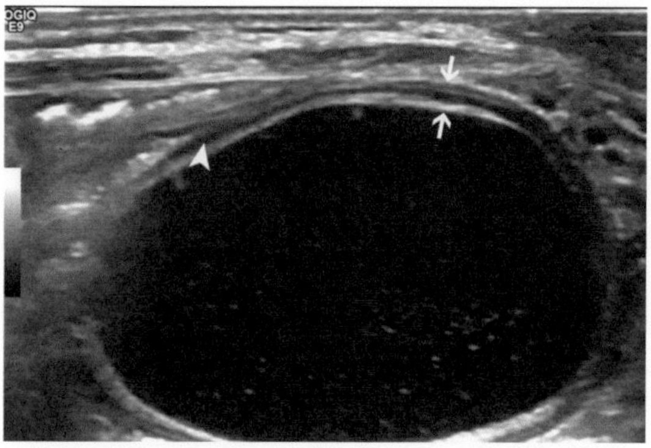

Fig. 10.5 Ileal duplication cyst. Short-axis scan through the lower abdomen, to right of the midline, shows an anechoic mass with a hyperechoic inner mucosal layer and a hyperechoic outer muscular layer ("gut signature") (arrows). Note the common muscle tonaca between the duplication and the wall of the intestinal loop ("Y" sign) (arrowhead)

abdominal distension, constipation, intussusception, volvulus, and partial intestinal obstruction; ileal cysts may be asymptomatic or manifest with abdominal pain, small bowel obstruction, a palpable abdominal mass, or rectal bleeding (hematochezia). In rare cases, malignant transformation may occur in cysts containing heterotopic gastric mucosa [7]. Early diagnosis is important to avoid complications. Diagnosis is achieved through ultrasound and/or contrast studies, which can reveal a filling defect. Ultrasound can detect a cystic lesion with internal echoes or debris and show a characteristic double-layer appearance of the wall, with a hyperechoic inner mucosal layer and a hyperechoic outer muscular layer, known as the "gut signature" (Fig. 10.5). However, in cases complicated by inflammation, this sign may be less evident [1]. In the presence of a cystic mass near the intestine, the possibility of a duplication cyst should be considered. CT and MRI can be useful in defining the location and size of the cyst. Treatment typically involves surgical removal.

10.5 Malrotation

Intestinal malrotation, more accurately defined as "incomplete rotation," represents an anomaly of the normal process of rotation of the primitive intestine during fetal life [1, 8]. The intestine typically undergoes a 270° rotation around the axis of the superior mesenteric artery (SMA) in a counterclockwise direction, positioning the duodenojejunal junction in the left hypochondrium, to the left of the spine, and the cecum in the right iliac fossa. This arrangement creates an extended mesenteric root that effectively supports the small intestine [1].

In cases of malrotation, there is an interruption of the normal rotation that can occur at any point in the process, resulting in a shortening of the mesenteric root. This condition can be associated with a wide variety of symptoms ranging from chronic intestinal disturbances, with episodes of recurrent vomiting and abdominal distension, to acute abdominal pain with bilious vomiting, presenting as an abdominal emergency known as "volvulus" [9].

Currently, ultrasound has taken on an important role in the diagnosis of malrotation, proving to be comparable to contrast radiography in many cases. Specifically, during the ultrasound examination, the following feature should be assessed: the inversion of the normal anatomical relationships between the superior mesenteric artery (SMA) and the superior mesenteric vein (SMV), where the SMV is located to the left of the SMA (Fig. 10.6). The presence of this alteration should be sought not only cranially but also as caudally as possible, as it can occur more distally.

However, the absence of inversion of the positions of the superior mesenteric vessels does not exclude the presence of malrotation [1].

Visualination of these signs is not always straightforward due to the frequent presence of

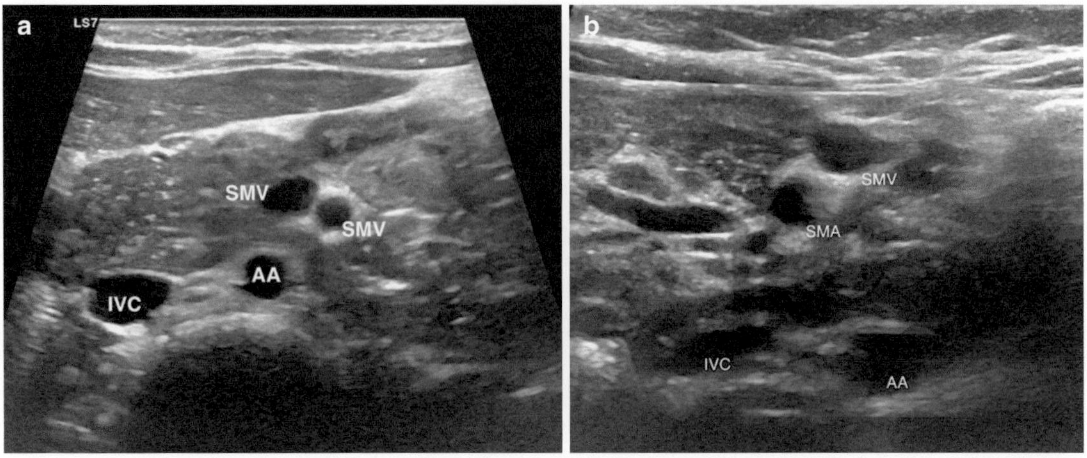

Fig. 10.6 (**a**) Transverse scan shows the normal relationships between the superior mesenteric artery (SMA) and the superior mesenteric vein (SMV). The vein is correctly located to the right of the artery. (**b**) Transverse scan shows the altered relationship between the SMA and SMV. The vein is inverted to the left of the artery. AA abdominal aorta, IV C inferior vena cava

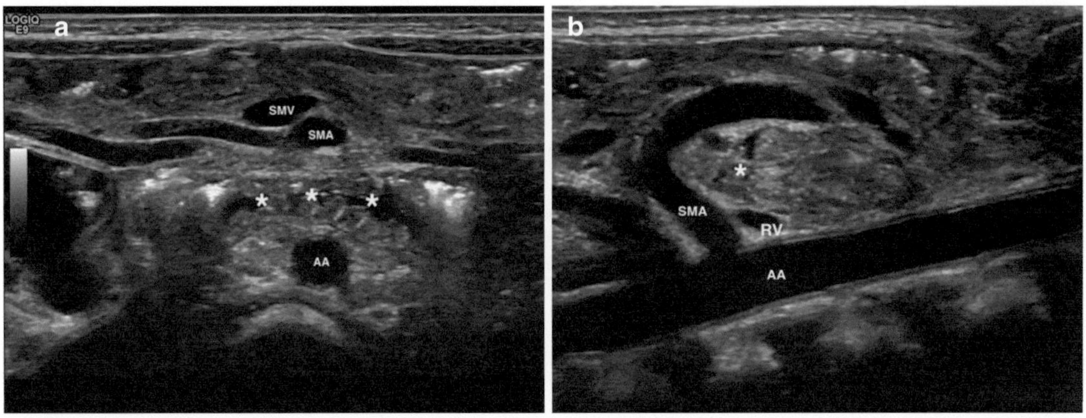

Fig. 10.7 (**a**) Transverse scan shows the D3 segment of the duodenum (*) in the retro-mesenteric space between the aorta and the superior mesenteric artery, crossing the vertebral column. (**b**) Longitudinal scan, B-mode, showing the aortomesenteric angle with passage into the D3 segment of the duodenum (*) and the left renal vein (RV). AA abdominal aorta, SMA superior mesenteric artery, SMV superior mesenteric vein

significant intestinal gas in neonates. Therefore, it is necessary to use gradual pressure with the probe to attempt to displace the air, or the patient can be positioned in the right lateral decubitus position, thereby facilitating the passage of fluid into the duodenum.

Additionally, the identification of the D3 segment of the duodenum in the retro-mesenteric space between the aorta and the SMA, crossing the vertebral column, with the duodenojejunal junction in the left hypochondrium allows the exclusion of the presence of malrotation (Fig. 10.7) [1, 9].

10.6 Volvulus

The term "midgut volvulus" refers to the twisting of the entire small intestine around the axis of the superior mesenteric artery, which can lead to obstruction and subsequent intestinal ischemia and necrosis. This condition occurs in patients with malrotation and primarily affects neonates, with onset in more than 90% of cases occurring within the first 3 months of life.

The pathognomonic ultrasound sign of this condition is the "Whirlpool sign" (Fig. 10.8).

The "Whirlpool sign" is more easily identifiable with the aid of color Doppler, which consists of the spiraling of the small intestine's mesentery and the superior mesenteric vein around the SMA, resulting in partial or total reduction of intestinal vascularization [1, 9].

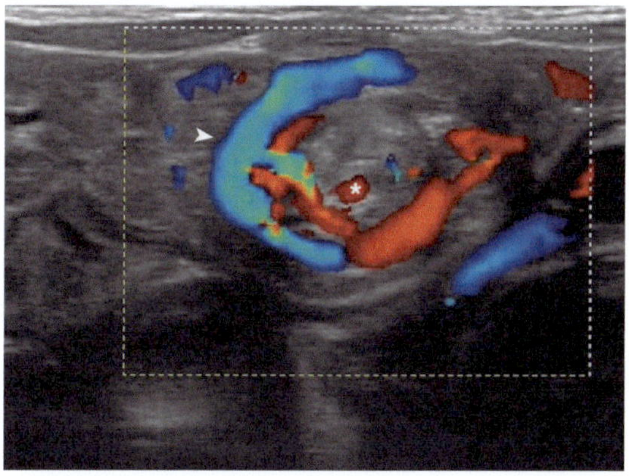

Fig. 10.8 Whirlpool sign. Axial scan, color Doppler US, shows small bowel volvulus with spiraling of the superior mesenteric vein (arrowhead) around the axis of the superior mesenteric artery (*)

10.7 Intestinal Polyp

In pediatric patients, 90% of gastrointestinal polyps are colorectal. These can be hamartomas or adenomas, but the most common type is the solitary juvenile polyp, which is most frequently located in the rectosigmoid region. This is a hamartoma characterized by a cystic component due to mucus retention secondary to obstruction of the mucous gland orifices [10, 11].

The most common presenting symptom is bright red rectal bleeding, which can lead to the development of anemia over time.

On ultrasound examination, it appears as an intraluminal nodular protrusion, measuring approximately 1–5 cm, typically pedunculated and mushroom-shaped, with evidence of adjacent anechoic cystic areas. On color Doppler examination, it shows rich intralesional vascularization with a well-defined vascular peduncle (Fig. 10.9) [1, 10, 11]. According to recent studies, in cases with very suggestive clinical features but negative conventional ultrasound, it is useful to perform the ultrasound examination after administering a contrast agent via the anal route [10].

Caution is needed for differential diagnosis with inflammatory pseudopolyps, which are typical of chronic inflammatory diseases. Unlike ham-

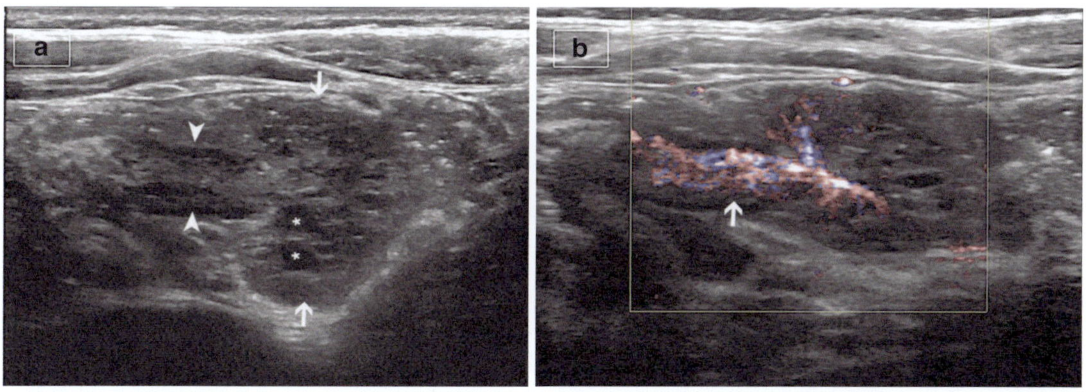

Fig. 10.9 Longitudinal scans. (**a**) Image shows a colon polyp that appears as a rounded nodular structure (arrows) with sharp margins and heterogeneous echostructure characterized by small anechoic cystic formations (*). The peduncle of the polyp can be identified (arrowhead). (**b**) Power Doppler image shows intralesional vascularization (arrow)

artomatous polyps, inflammatory pseudopolyps are more hyperechoic, are associated with thickening of the intestinal wall, and, importantly, do not present a vascular peduncle [11].

10.8 Omental Infarction

Omental infarction is a rare cause of acute abdomen in children and is caused by torsion or thrombosis of the omental panniculus, resulting in reduced vascularization and ischemia. It can be primary, with no evident cause, or secondary to trauma or other abdominal conditions such as omental adhesions, inguinal hernias, cysts, or tumors [12].

In most cases, the right segment of the greater omentum is involved, which is longer, heavier, and more mobile than the left segment. The main risk factor is obesity, which leads to increased deposition of perivascular fat, resulting in reduced blood supply to the growing omentum and an increase in its weight, facilitating the onset of torsion or traction on the more distal portions.

On ultrasound examination, it appears as an oval hyperechoic mass, typically located in the subhepatic region, anchored to the abdominal wall, with no evidence of internal vascularization on color Doppler examination (Fig. 10.10) [1, 12].

An important characteristic that facilitates the recognition of omental infarction is its adhesion to the anterior abdominal wall (Fig. 10.11), which results in the absence of movement during respiratory efforts [12]. This feature, known as the "tethered fat sign," can be evaluated using M-mode, which shows a linear laminar pattern both at the level of the superficial tissue and in the underlying omental tissue, delineating the typical immobile appearance referred to as the "barcode sign" (Fig. 10.12) [13, 14].

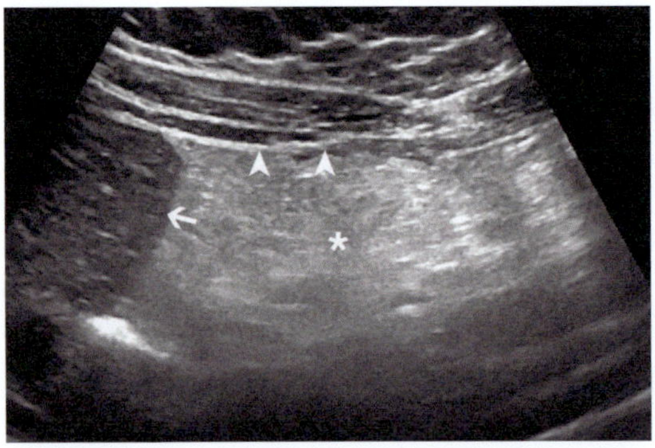

Fig. 10.10 Omental infarction. Transverse scan shows a hyperechoic oval mass (*) located in the right upper abdominal quadrant, below the lower hepatic border (arrow), just behind the anterior abdominal wall (arrowheads)

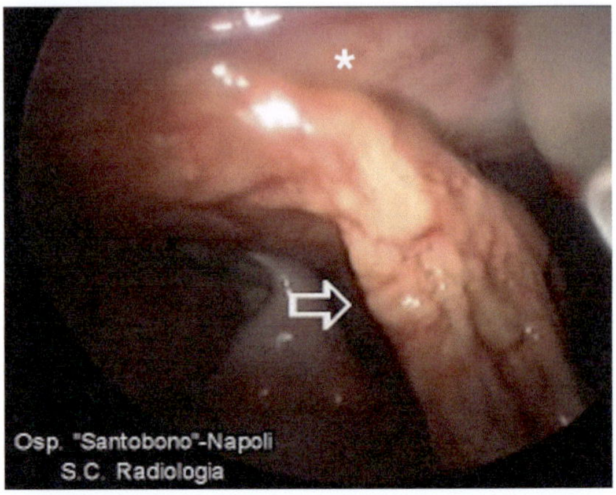

Fig. 10.11 Laparoscopy. Omental tissue (arrow) tethered to the abdominal wall (*)

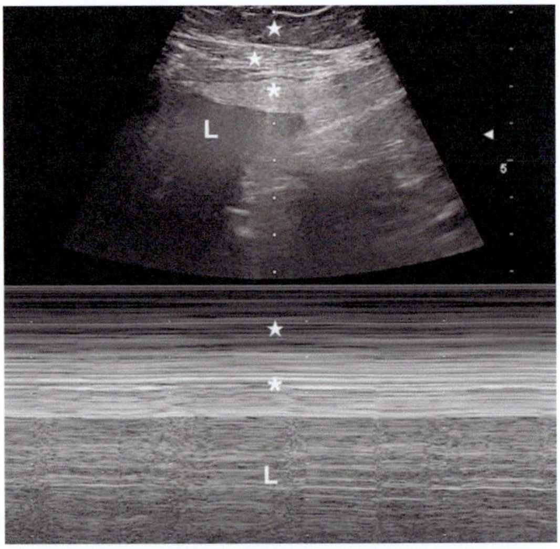

Fig. 10.12 "Tethered fat sign." Longitudinal scan. A subhepatic mass (*) is tethered to the abdominal wall (stars) and then displayed motionless on M-mode. The M-mode demonstrates a linear pattern in both mental fat and superficial tissue. This pattern is already known as the "barcode sign" or "stratosphere sign." L liver

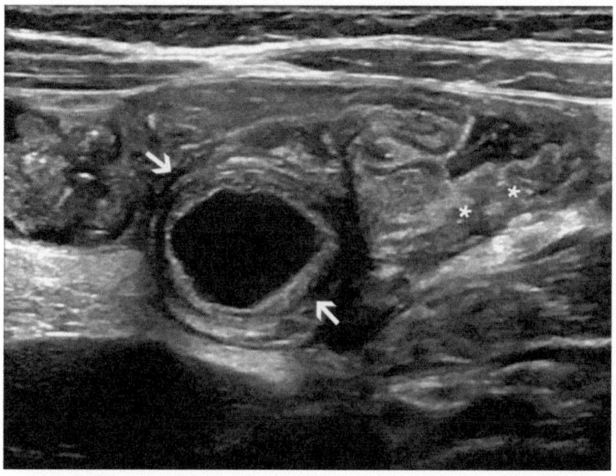

Fig. 10.13 Meckel's diverticulum. The Image shows a fluid-distended, blind-ending loop (arrows), connected to the small bowel (*)

10.9 Meckel's Diverticulum

This is the most common structural congenital anomaly of the gastrointestinal tract and arises from the fibrous degeneration of the umbilical end of the omphalomesenteric duct, occurring near the distal ileum. About 2% of the population has a Meckel's diverticulum, and it usually presents with complications in the early years of life [15].

It originates from the antimesenteric border of the small intestine, often about 60 cm from the ileocecal valve, and can reach a length of 5 cm with a diameter of up to 2 cm. On ultrasound examination, it appears as a blind-ending peristaltic loop connected to the small bowel (Fig. 10.13) [1, 16].

References

1. Esposito F, Di Serafino M, Mercogliano C, et al. The pediatric gastrointestinal tract: ultrasound findings in acute diseases. J Ultrasound. 2019;22(4):409–22. https://doi.org/10.1007/s40477-018-00355-0.
2. van Wassenaer EA, de Voogd FAE, van Rijn RR, et al. Bowel ultrasound measurements in healthy children – systematic review and meta-analysis. Pediatr Radiol. 2020;50(4):501–8. https://doi.org/10.1007/s00247-019-04567-2.
3. Indiran V, Selvaraj V. The cervix sign and other sonographic signs of hypertrophic pyloric stenosis. Abdom Radiol (NY). 2016;41(10):2085–6. https://doi.org/10.1007/s00261-016-0809-5.
4. Yousef A, Daneman A, Amirabadi A, Faingold R. The impact of high-frequency transducers on the sonographic measurements of the pyloric muscle thickness in infants. Pediatr Radiol. 2024;54(5):737–42. https://doi.org/10.1007/s00247-024-05881-0.
5. Li XZ, Wang H, Song J, Liu Y, Lin YQ, Sun ZX. Ultrasonographic diagnosis of intussusception in children: a systematic review and meta-analysis. J Ultrasound Med. 2021;40(6):1077–84. https://doi.org/10.1002/jum.15504.
6. Esposito F, Ambrosio C, De Fronzo S, et al. Fluoroscopy-guided hydrostatic reduction of intussusception in infancy: role of pharmacological premedication. Radiol Med. 2015;120(6):549–56. https://doi.org/10.1007/s11547-014-0486-9.
7. Sangüesa Nebot C, et al. Enteric duplication cysts in children: varied presentations, varied imaging findings. Insights Imaging. 2018;9(6):1097–106. https://doi.org/10.1007/s13244-018-0660-z.
8. McCurdie FK, Meshaka R, Leung G, et al. Ultrasound for infantile midgut malrotation: techniques, pearls, and pitfalls. Pediatr Radiol. 2024;54:2099–111. https://doi.org/10.1007/s00247-024-06067-4.
9. Yang X, Wang W, Wang K, Zhao J, Sun L, Jiang S, Wang Y, Feng W, Ding G, Fu T, Li A, Geng L. Identification and treatment of intestinal malrotation with midgut volvulus in childhood: a multicenter retrospective study. Front Pediatr. 2024;12:1390856. https://doi.org/10.3389/fped.2024.1390856. PMID: 38803636; PMCID: PMC11128588.
10. Zhang M, Lin H, Hu J, Jing XX, Qin LL. The value of colorectal filling contrast ultrasonography in diagnosing pediatric juvenile polyps. J Clin Ultrasound. 2022;50(4):564–72. https://doi.org/10.1002/jcu.23198. Epub 2022 Mar 22. PMID: 35318682.
11. Zhang Y, Li SX, Xie LM, Shi B, Ju H, Bai YZ, Zhang SC. Sonographic diagnosis of juvenile polyps in children. Ultrasound Med Biol. 2012;38(9):1529–33. https://doi.org/10.1016/j.ultrasmedbio.2012.05.018. Epub 2012 Jul 3. PMID: 22766117.
12. Esposito F, Ferrara D, Schillirò ML, Grillo A, Diplomatico M, Tomà P. "Tethered fat sign": the sonographic sign of omental infarction. Ultrasound Med Biol. 2020;46(5):1105–10. https://doi.org/10.1016/j.ultrasmedbio.2020.01.003. Epub 2020 Feb 5. PMID: 32035686.
13. Esposito F, Ferrara D, D'Auria D, Gaglione G, Diplomatico M, Noviello D, Zeccolini M, Tomà P. M-mode ultrasound for assessment of the "tethered fat sign" in children: an easily performed way to certify a dynamic process as a still picture. Quant Imaging Med Surg. 2024;14(6):4134–40. https://doi.org/10.21037/qims-23-1691. Epub 2024 May 24. PMID: 38846297; PMCID: PMC11151229.
14. Esposito F, Di Serafino M, Mauro A, Mercogliano C, Cocco C, Zenzeri L, Ferrara D, Iacobellis F, Evangelisti M, Ziparo C, Di Nardo G. Not only

fat: omental infarction and its mimics in children. Clinical and ultrasound findings: a pictorial review. J Ultrasound. 2020;23(4):621–9. https://doi.org/10.1007/s40477-020-00492-5. Epub 2020 Jul 4. PMID: 32623635; PMCID: PMC7588577.
15. Levy A, Hobbs C. From the archives of the AFIP. Meckel diverticulum: radiologic features with pathologic correlation. Radiographics. 2004;24(2):565–87. https://doi.org/10.1148/rg.242035187.
16. Farrell MB. Meckel's diverticulum imaging. J Nucl Med Technol. 2020;48(3):189–90. https://doi.org/10.2967/jnmt.120.244137.

Serendipity Encounters at Bowel Ultrasound Examination in IBD Patients

11

Fulvia Terracciano, Antonella Marra, Veronica Nassisi, Angelo Andriulli, and Ilario de Sio

11.1 Clinical Case 1: When the Ultrasound Acts as a Fishing Net

A 56-year-old man with a 10-year history of ulcerative colitis (UC) was admitted to the emergency department complaining of abdominal pain and melena. The patient had been on mesalazine since the initial manifestation of the disease but did not undergo follow-up evaluations being symptomless. He reported having a brother with the same condition. On admission, the patient was hemodynamically stable, and his laboratory tests revealed moderate anemia, along with a slight increase in inflammatory markers. He also reported recent flu-like symptoms.

As part of the diagnostic workup, the patient underwent a gastroscopy, which was negative, ruling out upper gastrointestinal bleeding. To further investigate the potential source, a colonoscopy and intestinal ultrasound (IUS) were scheduled on the same day. AT IUS investigation, performed after bowel preparation with macrogol, the right colon appeared moderately distended with fluid (Fig. 11.1), though the colonic wall maintained a preserved haustral pattern. An unexpected echogenic intraluminal lesion was appreciated to originate from the posterior wall of the colon which proved difficult to discriminate between a solid mass and fecal residue on B-mode evaluation.

Consequently, a contrast-enhanced ultrasound (CEUS) was performed to further clarify the findings (Figs. 11.2 and 11.3; Video 11.1).

On CEUS the echogenic mass was found to have a hypervascular pattern in all phases, confirming its solid nature; the picture discharged the assumption of fecal residue. The subsequent, same-day colonoscopy documented the presence of a large colonic polyp with a long stalk which was entirely removed (Fig. 11.4 and 11.11, 11.13, and 11.14).

Supplementary Information The online version contains supplementary material available at https://doi.org/10.1007/978-3-032-11418-1_11. The videos can be accessed individually by clicking the DOI link in the accompanying figure caption or by scanning this link with the SN More Media App.

F. Terracciano (✉) · A. Andriulli
Division of Gastroenterology and Digestive Endoscopy, Fondazione IRCCS "Casa Sollievo della Sofferenza", San Giovanni Rotondo, Italy

A. Marra
National Institute of Gastroenterology, IRCCS "Saverio de Bellis" Research Hospital, Castellana Grotte, Italy
e-mail: antonella.marra@irccsdebellis.it

V. Nassisi
General Medicine Unit, "Casa di Cura San Camillo", Messina, Italy

I. de Sio
Gastroenterology Unit, Department of Clinical Medicine and Surgery, University L. Vanvitelli, Naples, Italy

F. Terracciano et al. (eds.), *Bowel Ultrasound Compared with Endoscopy*,
https://doi.org/10.1007/978-3-032-11418-1_11

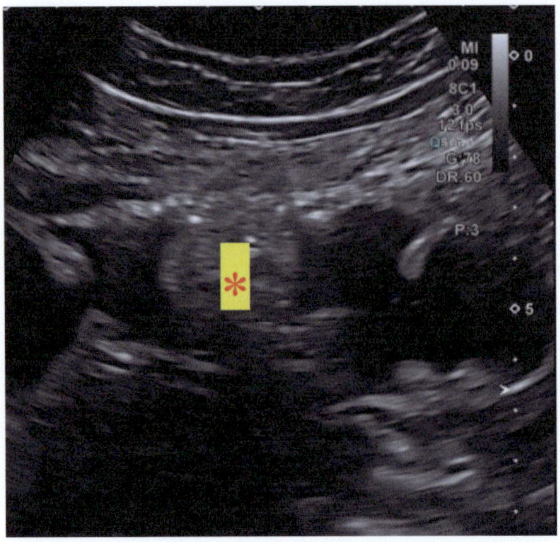

Fig. 11.1 Echogenic solid colonic lesion arising from the posterior wall (asterisk)

Comment Clearly, this represents a case of serendipity encounter at US bowel investigation. It is well established that ultrasound is not a standard screening method for detecting lesions arising from the colonic wall [2]. However, in this case, the combination of fluid-induced distension of the colon, the size of the polyp, and the use of contrast-enhanced ultrasound (CEUS) allowed us to identify it prior to the scheduled colonoscopy.

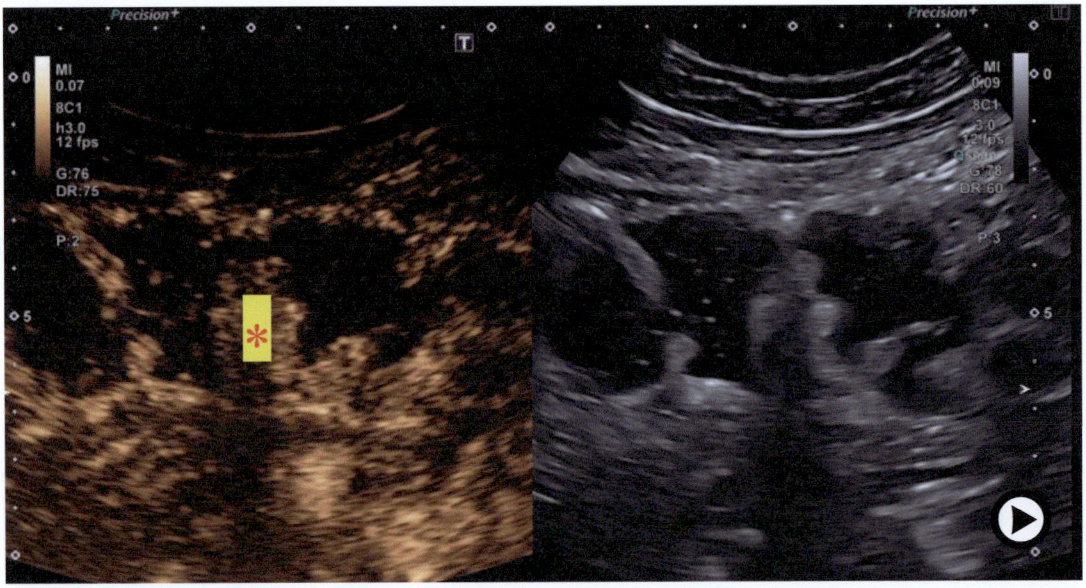

Fig. 11.2 CEUS arterial phase: the echogenic mass proved hypervascular (asterisk) Video 11.1 On CEUS the echogenic mass was found to have a hypervascular pattern in all phases, confirming its solid nature (▶ https://doi.org/10.1007/000-j31)

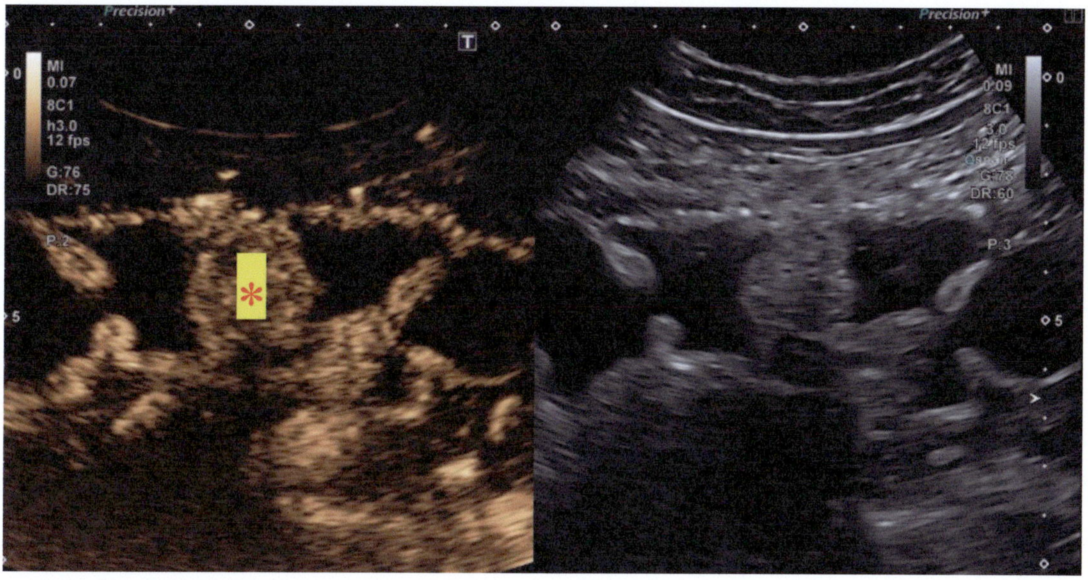

Fig. 11.3 CEUS late phase: the mass remains vascularized (asterisk)

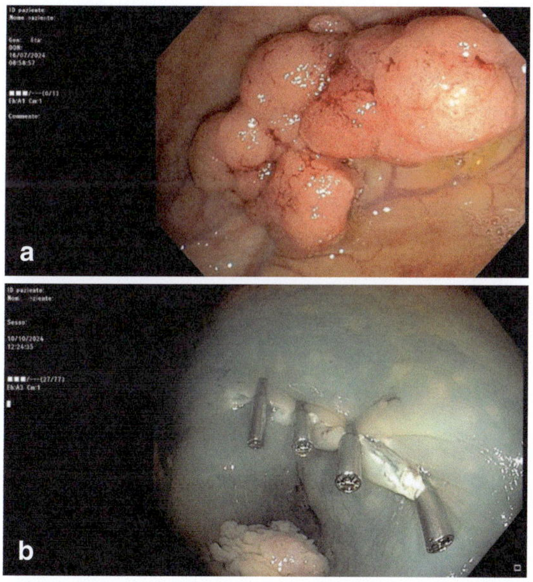

Fig. 11.4 (**a**) Granular, mixed nodular type, laterally spreading tumor (LST-G MN, 0-Is + IIa according Paris Classification). (**b**) Appearance of scar after complete resection and endoclips placement

11.2 Clinical Case 2: A Rare Case of Sigmoid Colon Obstruction in a Woman

A 41-year-old primiparous woman experienced an acute flare of ulcerative colitis 9 years prior to the present and has been on maintenance therapy with 5-ASA and azathioprine since then. At the age of 18, she underwent a surgery for the removal of an ovarian cyst. The histological diagnosis was of ovarian endometriosis. Two weeks before actual presentation, she began to complain of abdominal cramps in the lower abdomen and obstinate constipation which could not be managed with common laxatives; the symptoms had not been previously experienced by the patient.

On physical inspection, the abdomen was distended, tender, and tympanitic on percussion with high-pitched bowel sounds. Routine blood chemistry was normal. A colonoscopic examination documented at about 20 cm from the anal verge a submucosal lesion partially occupying the colonic lumen with a normal-appearing mucosal pattern. The colon appeared rigid in that area which prevented further inspection of the organ (Fig. 11.5). Histology showed no inflammatory changes consistent with active disease, thus confirming a likely submucosal cause for the obstruction. Submucosal lesion occluding the sigmoid lumen was confirmed by normal histologic pattern of colonic biopsies. On transabdominal ultrasound, a 17-mm hypoechoic lesion was observed originating from the submucosal layer, causing narrowing of the sigmoid lumen (Fig. 11.6). Ultrasound scan of the remaining intestinal tract showed no coarse masses or wall thickening, neither lymphadenopathy nor mesenteric reactions. A follow-up transabdominal ultrasound performed 15 days later showed persistence of the hypoechoic wall-thickening lesion in the sigmoid colon, although it had decreased in size (11 mm in diameter) (Fig. 11.7)). MRI confirmed the presence of a hypo-isointense oval lesion, measuring approximately 15 × 17 mm, at the level of the sigmoid colon (Fig. 11.8). After informed consent was signed, a transabdominal ultrasound-guided biopsy of the lesion with a needle Biomol 18 G 15 mm was performed. The post-procedure was uneventful. At histology a fibrous tissue with glands coated with cylindrical epithelium and surrounded by spindle cell stroma was observed. The glands' nuclei were positive for estrogen and progesterone (Fig. 11.9, immunoblotting with anti-progesterone receptor). The stroma was positive for CD10 (Fig. 11.10, Hematoxylin–eosin magnification 20×). The histologic diagnosis was compatible with endometriosis. Therapy with danazol was instituted.

Comment Endometriosis is a chronic and recurrent disease characterized by proliferation of endometrial tissue outside the uterine cavity. The incidence of bowel involvement has been reported to vary from 3% to 34% of cases. The true incidence of endometriosis causing bowel obstruction is unknown, although complete obstruction of the bowel lumen occurs in less than 1% of cases.

Intestinal endometriosis usually manifests itself as asymptomatic small serosal implants. Under hormonal influence, these implants may proliferate and bleed cyclically, causing symptoms such as crampy abdominal pain, tenesmus, abdominal distension, diarrhea, vomiting, rectal pain, infertility, abdominal mass, increased urinary frequency, constipation, or hematochezia. Acute, partial, or complete bowel obstruction has also been reported, but its frequency is rare.

The diagnosis of intestinal endometriosis should be considered in any premenopausal woman who complains of gastrointestinal symptoms, especially when these symptoms occur cyclically and associated with endometriosis implants in other sites. However, most cases are found accidentally at surgery. Imaging studies

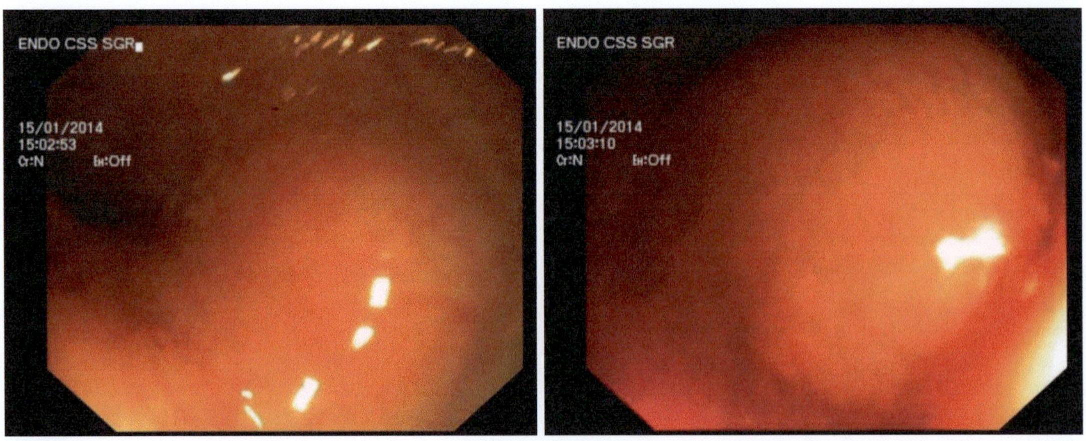

Fig. 11.5 Submucosal colonic lesion covered by normal-appearing mucosa

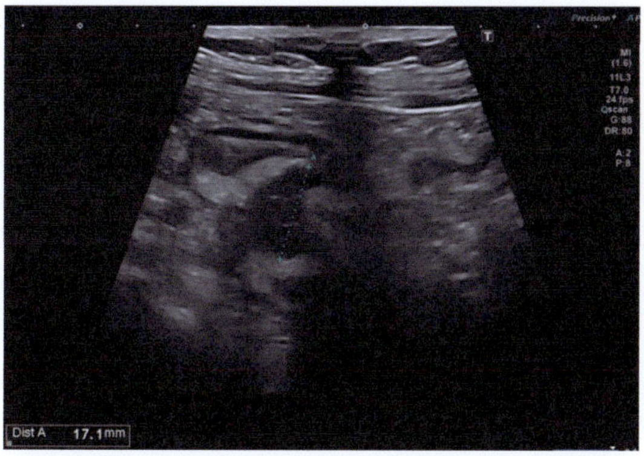

Fig. 11.6 Hypoechoic lesion (max diameter 17 mm) that seems to originate from the submucosa, occluding the sigmoid lumen

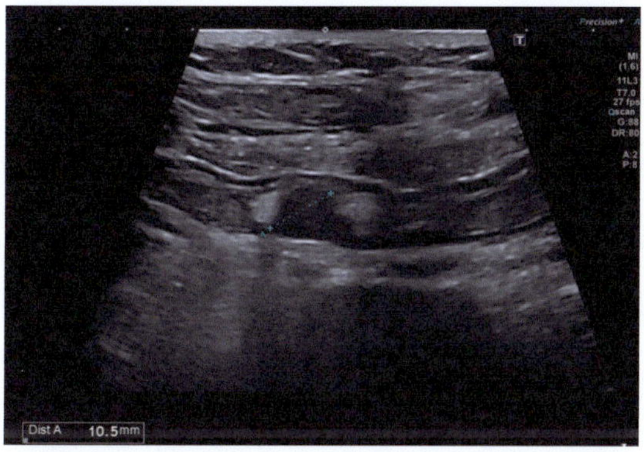

Fig. 11.7 Longitudinal scan of the sigmoid colon shows the known hypoechoic lesion with well-defined margins, in continuity with the intestinal wall

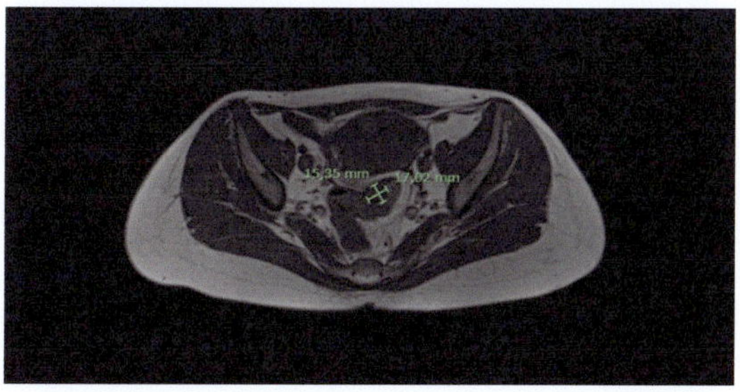

Fig. 11.8 Hypo-isointense oval lesion measuring approximately 15 × 17 mm within the sigma wall

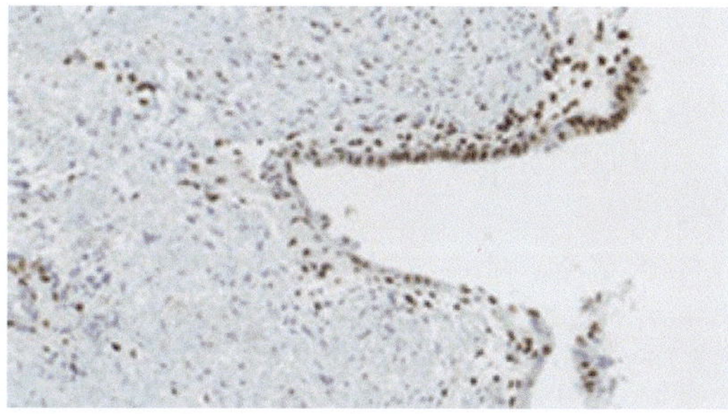

Fig. 11.9 Fibrous tissue within glands coated with cylindrical epithelium, surrounded by spindle cell stroma. The glands' nuclei were positive for estrogen and progesterone

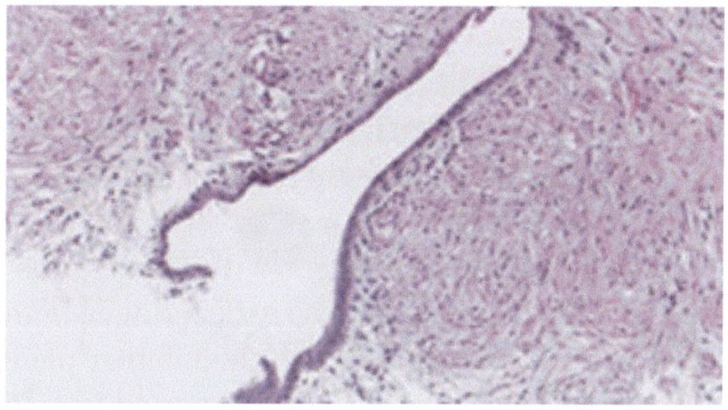

Fig. 11.10 Hematoxylin–eosin magnification ×20. Stroma was positive for CD10

such as multislice computed tomography (CT) (especially if combined with enteroclysis), MRI, endoscopic ultrasound, and transvaginal sonography have potential for detecting the condition.

Similar to the presented case, colonoscopy has not proved helpful in diagnosis, but recommended in all patients with suspected endometriosis to rule out mucosal involvement and malignant lesions. Despite this array of diagnostic methods, laparoscopy remains the only investigation able to confirm the presence of intestinal endometriosis. Transabdominal ultrasound is not sensitive enough for diagnosis.

Many studies have shown that the ultrasound-guided fine-needle biopsy/cytology of abdominal lesions is simple, relatively painless, reasonably safe, accurate, time saving, and a reliable method to obtain specimen for specific histologic/cytologic diagnosis, with less trauma, minimal discomfort, and low complication rate [3].

The present report points out that endometriosis remains a challenging condition for clinicians. In a woman of childbearing age presenting with intestinal obstruction and more common conditions excluded, a high level of suspicion of endometriosis should be maintained.

Below we present ultrasound images of a further case of intestinal endometriosis (Fig. 11.11).

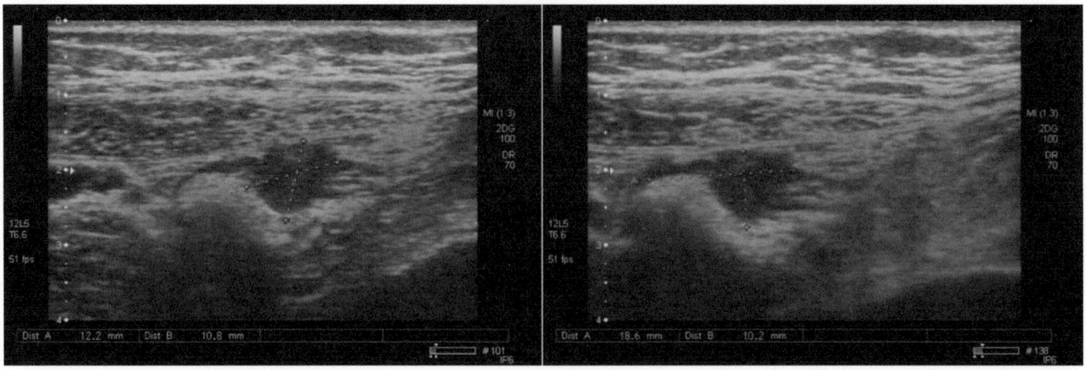

Fig. 11.11 Longitudinal scan of the colon shows a well-defined hypoechoic lesion adjacent to the colonic wall, measuring 18 × 10 mm

11.3 Clinical Case 3: May the Appendix Resurge After Appendectomy?

A 25-year-old female patient with Crohn's disease presented to the emergency department with a two-day history of primarily abdominal pain, initially located around the umbilicus and later to the right lower quadrant. Anorexia and nausea were also disturbing the patient. Her surgical history included an appendectomy 10 years ago. Her axillary temperature was 37.5 °C, blood pressure 125/70 mmHg, heart rate 76 beats/min, and respiratory rate 16 breaths/min. Abdominal examination revealed tenderness and guarding in the right lower quadrant at palpation. Routine laboratory tests showed normal electrolyte panels and blood cells, at exception of white blood cell count of 12,000/μL. Urinalysis was unremarkable. In the suspicion of a flare-up of the disease or of one of its complications, a gastroenterologic consultation was scheduled. At the requested ultrasound a heterogeneous hypo-anechoic mass of 20 × 10 mm in size (Fig. 11.12a–c; Video 11.2) in contact with the cecum was appreciated with a mild hypertrophy of the surrounding mesentery. The terminal ileum was not thickened and there were no images of sinus or abscess collections. A presumptive diagnosis of inflammation of the appendiceal stump was made. The CT scan of the abdomen and pelvis showed a tubular structure that extended from the cecum, with an enlarged wall consistent with an inflamed appendiceal stump. Antibiotic therapy led to the clinical and laboratory resolutions.

Comment Stump appendicitis is a rare delayed complication of appendectomy, the incidence of which remains unknown. The condition is thought to be underreported in the literature. A long residual appendiceal stump is a recognized risk factor for stump appendicitis. The length of the stump ranges from 0.5 to 6.5 cm [4]. Mangi and Berger [5] suggested that leaving an appendiceal stump of less than 3 mm in depth with visualization of the appendiceal base can minimize the incidence of stump appendicitis. Laparoscopic appendectomy is now a widely accepted surgical technique for treating appendicitis and its growing use may increase the frequency of stump appendicitis due to the potential limitations of the technique such as smaller field of vision, lack of three-dimensional perspective, and absence of tactile feedback, all issues that might occur in thus leaving a longer stump after surgery [6].

The wide spectrum of pathologies included in the differential diagnosis for right lower quadrant pain in patients with a history of appendectomy can often delay the diagnosis and treatment of

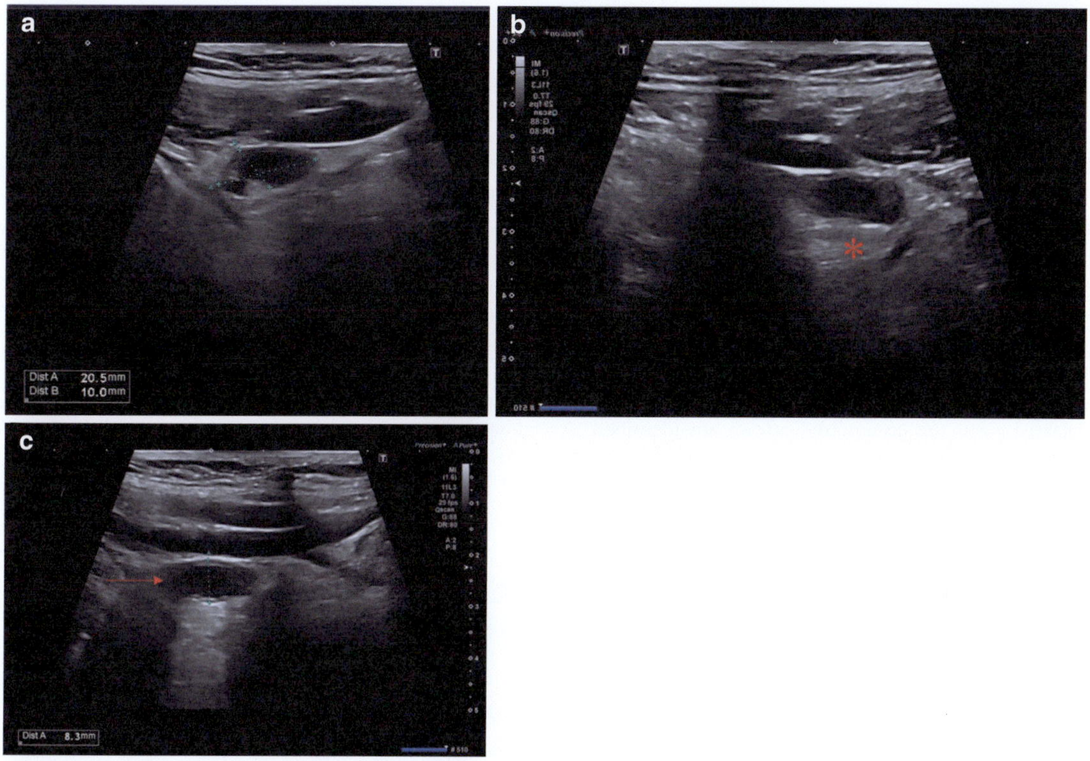

Fig. 11.12 Scan of the right iliac fossa using a linear probe. (**a**) A hypo-anechoic tubular lesion measuring 20 × 10 mm is detected at the site of the previous appendectomy. (**b**) It appears as a blind-ending tubular structure surrounded by mild mesenteric hypertrophy (*). (**c**) It has a thin wall and its content appears to be fluid, as confirmed by the presence of posterior acoustic enhancement (red arrow)

stump appendicitis. In the present case, the ultrasound was able to exclude more common causes of abdominal pain in the right iliac fossa (such as relapse of Crohn's disease, urinary and gynecological causes) and to raise the suspicion of the condition, allowing the immediate start of conservative treatment.

Below we present ultrasound images of further cases of stumpitis (Figs. 11.13 and 11.14).

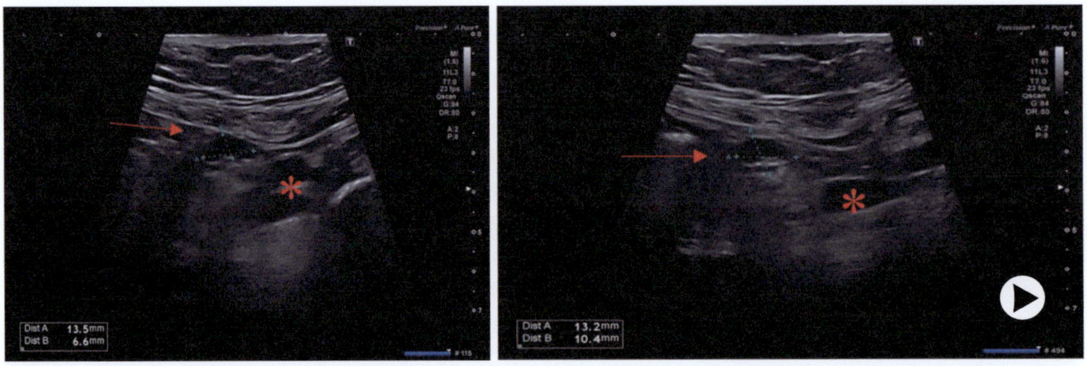

Fig. 11.13 Scan of the right iliac fossa. The iliac vessels (asterisk) and the cecum (red arrow) are identified. A tubular structure in continuity with the cecum is visualized, containing fluid and measuring 13 × 10 mmVideo 11.2 A hypo-anechoic tubular lesion detected at the site of the previous appendectomy; it appears as a blind-ending tubular structure surrounded by mild mesenteric hypertrophy, with a thin wall and its content appears to be fluid (▶ https://doi.org/10.1007/000-j30)

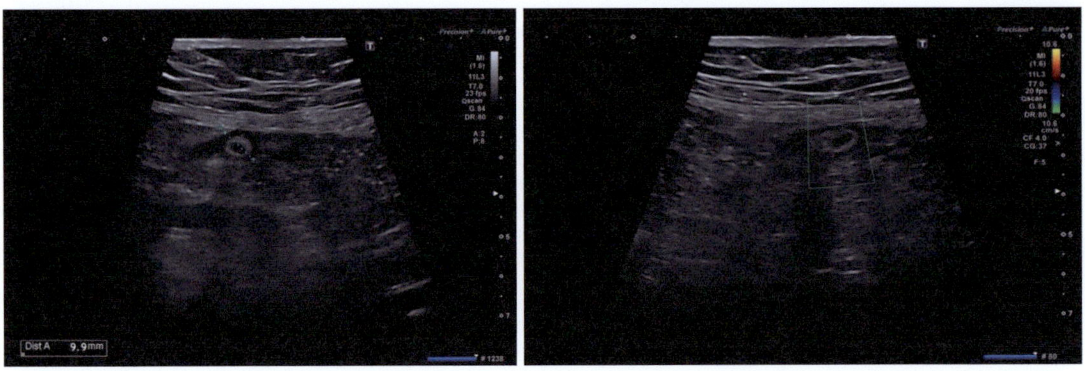

Fig. 11.14 Scan of the right iliac fossa in an appendectomized patient complaining of localized pain in that area. (**a**) Transverse section of the inflamed appendiceal stump measuring 10 mm. (**b**) No Doppler signal detected

11.4 Clinical Case 4: Doctor! Help Me! I Think I Have Appendicitis on the Left!

A 45-year-old male with a history of Ulcerative Colitis (UC) and obesity presented to the emergency department with a two-day history of sharp, stabbing, non-radiating pain localized to the left lower quadrant of the abdomen. The pain initially started in the periumbilical region and progressively moved to the left lower quadrant. Associated symptoms included nausea and anorexia but no fever, vomiting, or bowel disturbances.

The patient was alert, afebrile, and hemodynamically stable. Abdominal examination revealed mild guarding and tenderness localized to the left lower quadrant. Rebound tenderness was mildly positive, but no signs of peritonitis were observed. Bowel sounds were present, and the rest of the physical examination was unremarkable. Initial blood tests showed an elevated white blood cell (WBC) count of 13.5×10^9/L and a mildly elevated C-reactive protein (CRP) level of 11 mg/L (nv < 5). Liver and renal function tests were normal. Ultrasound was performed: the thickness of the colon was normal, which excluded a flare-up of the underlying ulcerative rectal disease; at the site of the pain, in the left iliac fossa, we identified a highly hyperechoic and heterogeneous area with ill-defined margins, which elicited marked tenderness upon probe pressure approximately 25 mm in lenght (Fig. 11.15; Video 11.3).

A contrast-enhanced computed tomography scan of the abdomen was performed to investigate further. The CT scan (Fig. 11.16) revealed an ill-defined, 25 mm ovoid lesion with fatty stranding in the anterior wall of the sigmoid colon, accompanied by reactive lymph nodes. These findings were consistent with epiploic appendagitis. On the right side the appendix was normal, ruling out appendicitis as the primary cause of the patient's symptoms.

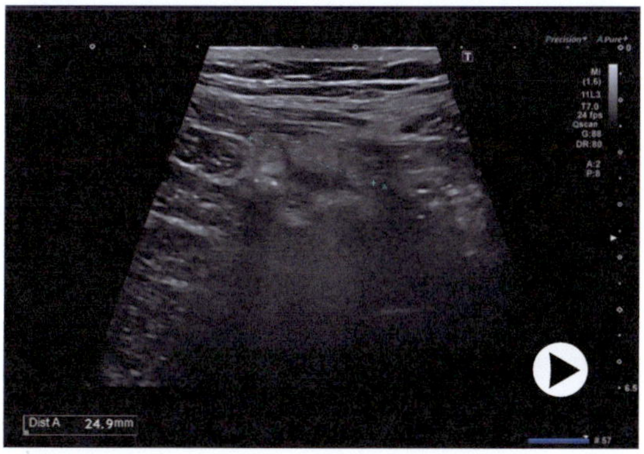

Fig. 11.15 A linear probe was positioned in the left iliac fossa at the point of maximal tenderness reported by the patient. A 25 mm heterogeneous hyperechoic area with ill-defined margins was observed adjacent to the sigmoid colonVideo 11.3 An heterogeneous hyperechoic area with ill-defined margins was observed adjacent to the sigmoid colon (▶ https://doi.org/10.1007/000-j32)

Given the self-limiting nature of the condition, conservative management was initiated. The patient was prescribed non-steroidal anti-inflammatory drugs (NSAIDs) to control pain and inflammation. No antibiotics or surgical intervention were required and there were no signs of complications, such as bowel obstruction or abscess formation. The patient was instructed about the benign course of the condition and the expected resolution of symptoms within 1–2 weeks. He was also advised to seek medical attention if symptoms worsened or new symptoms developed, such as fever or vomiting.

At the one-week follow-up, the patient reported significant improvement in symptoms, with pain decreasing in intensity. He was able to resume normal activities without difficulty. A follow up ultrasound check was performed, showing a reduction in the size of the ovoid lesion (length 18 mm, Fig. 11.17).

Comment Epiploic appendagitis, first described in 1956, is a rare condition often misdiagnosed due to its resemblance to other, more common causes of acute abdominal pain, such as appendicitis or diverticulitis [7]. Misdiagnosis can result in unnecessary hospital admissions, antibiotic treatments, or even surgery. However, since epiploic appendagitis is typically benign and self-limiting, early and accurate diagnosis is crucial. In this case, timely ultrasound followed by CT

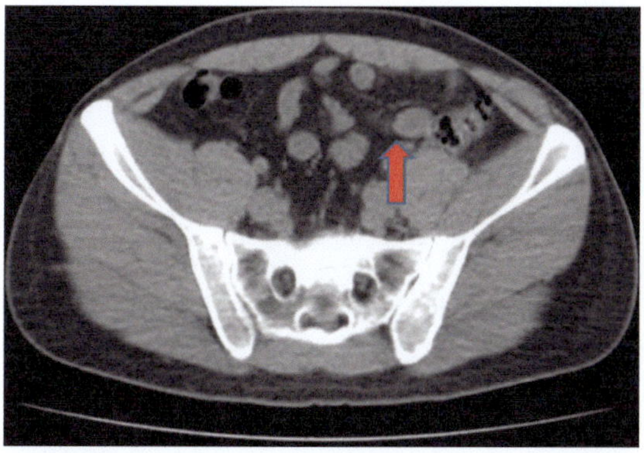

Fig. 11.16 CT scan: an ill-defined, 25 mm ovoid lesion with fatty stranding in the anterior wall of the sigmoid colon, accompanied by reactive lymph nodes was observed (red arrow)

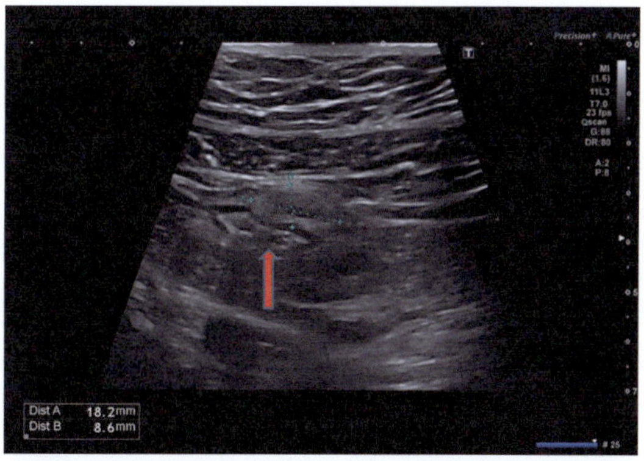

Fig. 11.17 Transverse scan of the sigmoid colon. The hyperechoic area has decreased in size (18 mm) and shows better-defined margins. A close relationship with the sigmoid colon is evident (red arrow)

imaging played a key role in confirming the diagnosis and avoiding unnecessary surgical procedures.

The pathophysiology of epiploic appendagitis involves either spontaneous torsion or venous thrombosis of the epiploic appendage, leading to ischemia, infarction, and localized peritonitis. This process results in aseptic fat necrosis, which accounts for the characteristic findings seen on imaging, such as fat stranding around an ovoid lesion [8].

Management of epiploic appendagitis is primarily conservative, consisting of anti-inflammatory medications for pain control and close monitoring. Surgery is rarely required and is reserved for complications, such as bowel obstruction or abscess formation. Most patients experience symptom resolution within 1–2 weeks [9].

11.5 Clinical Case 5: A Good Doctor with a Probe Is Better than Sherlock Holmes

A 29-year-old male patient with a known history of Crohn's disease, currently in clinical remission and on maintenance therapy with adalimumab, presented to our gastroenterology outpatient clinic for acute-onset, and severe central abdominal pain associated with nausea and vomiting. During a previous ED admission, an unenhanced CT scan revealed the presence of air-fluid levels. The patient was admitted to the short-stay observation unit for 48 hours, where he received symptomatic treatment with antispasmodic agents, with only partial clinical improvement. He was subsequently discharged with the recommendation to further gastroenterology follow-up visit, due to suspicion of a mild disease flare.

During our outpatient gastroenterological evaluation, the abdominal examination revealed a soft but tender abdomen in the mesogastric region, with preserved bowel peristalsis. Laboratory tests showed negative inflammatory markers and a normal complete blood count. Abdominal and intestinal ultrasound was also performed: in the region between the right flank and the mesogastrium, corresponding to the site of the referred pain, the normally regular intestinal wall—with a symmetrical and eucentric lumen—appeared interrupted by an irregular mural thickening, associated with mild surrounding mesenteric hypertrophy. For a more detailed assessment, we used a high-frequency linear probe: in that region, the bowel loop, likely the jejuno-ileal loop, exhibited marked wall thickening, with a maximum of 16 mm. Wall stratification was obscured completely and the lumen appeared eccentric. The loop was uncompressible under graded transducer pressure and with lack of intramural vascularity on color Doppler imaging (Fig. 11.18).

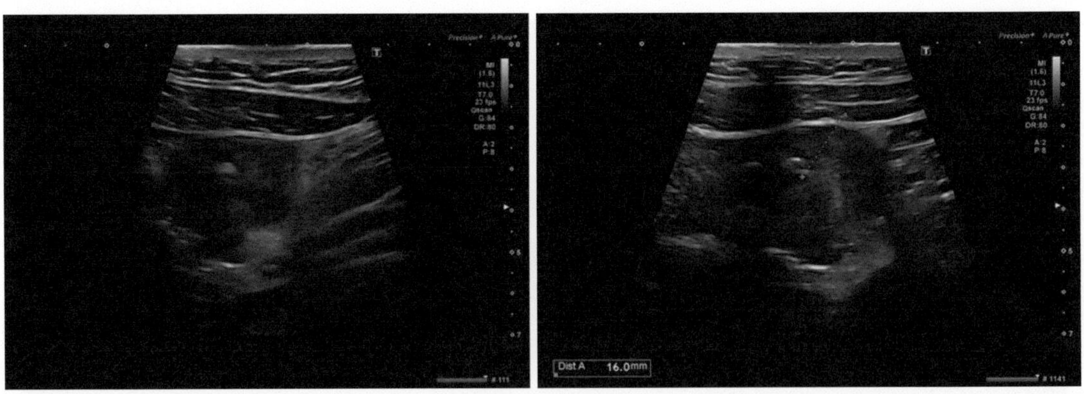

Fig. 11.18 Transverse section in the mesogastric region. A bowel loop is visualized with marked wall thickening (approximately 16 mm) and complete loss of wall stratification

The patient was admitted for further diagnostic workup. Repeat laboratory testing confirmed persistently negative inflammatory markers, with normal complete blood count and electrolyte levels. However, carcinoembryonic antigen (CEA) and carbohydrate antigen 19-9 (CA19-9) were elevated to 5 and 10 times the upper limit of normal, respectively. A contrast-enhanced CT scan (Fig. 11.19) was subsequently performed, confirming the presence of a 5 × 5 cm lesion involving the jejunal loops, characterized by arterial phase enhancement—raising strong suspicion for a neoplastic process.

Given the inaccessibility of the lesion via endoscopy, a percutaneous core needle biopsy was performed under imaging guidance (Fig. 11.20). At histology, a moderately differentiated adenocarcinoma of the jejunum was diagnosed. The patient underwent segmental jejunal resection.

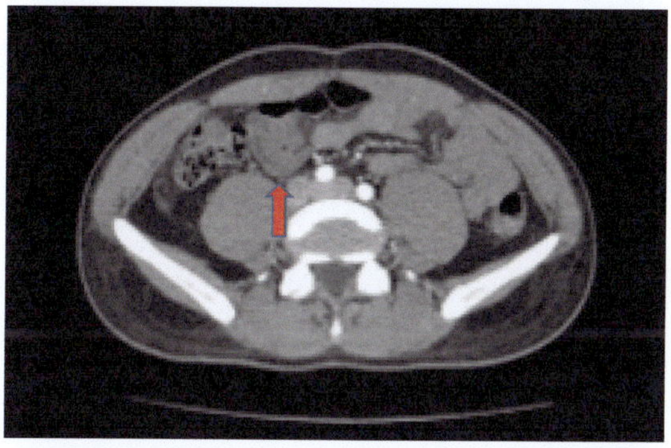

Fig. 11.19 CT scan: mesogastric region—a lesion involving the jejunal loops was identified, demonstrating arterial phase enhancement (red arrow)

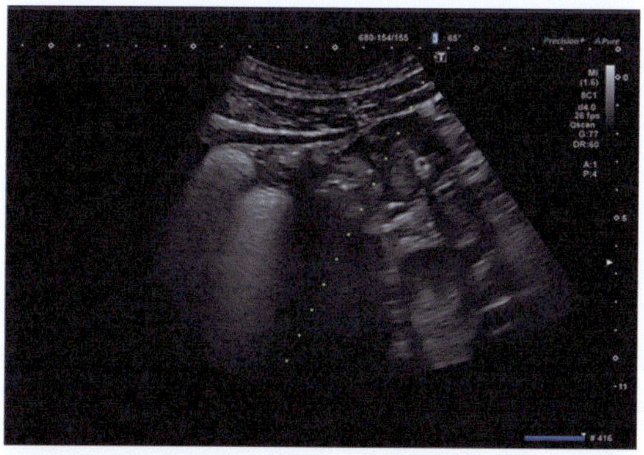

Fig. 11.20 Convex probe scan of the mesogastric region. Parietal thickening of a bowel loop is identified, with a dashed line indicating the planned needle trajectory for the upcoming percutaneous biopsy

Comment Small bowel cancer is a rare malignancy that comprises less than 5% of all gastrointestinal malignancies. The estimated annual incidence is 0.3–2.0 cases per 100,000 persons; it is most frequently diagnosed among people aged 55–64 [10]. Patients with inflammatory bowel diseases (IBD) are at significantly higher risk of small bowel adenocarcinomas than their non-IBD general populations, with Crohn's patients having at least a 12-fold increased risk and ulcerative colitis patients with a more controversial and modest two-fold increased risk compared to the general population [11].

Small bowel cancer has four common histological types: adenocarcinoma (30–40%), carcinoid tumor (35–42%), lymphoma (15–20%), and sarcoma (10–15%). Adenocarcinoma of the small bowel (SBA) is most commonly located in the duodenum (57%), while 29% of cases in the jejunum and 10% in the ileum. Clinical presentation of SBA is non-specific abdominal symptoms, such as abdominal pain, nausea, vomiting, gastrointestinal bleeding, and intestinal obstruction, which lead to an average delay of 6–10 months in diagnosis. Due to the rarity of this cancer, there have been no effective screening methods developed for SBA [12]. It is hypothesized that the SBA that occur in IBD patients are caused by chronically uncontrolled inflammation, as well as the long-term use of immunosuppressive agents. While chronic immunosuppression has been shown to promote carcinogenesis (e.g., the association of thiopurines with lymphomas and skin malignancies), there is no evidence linking any specific class of immunosuppressants to the risk of SBA [13]. The duration of small bowel CD is the most reliable risk factor for the development of SBA [11]. As described in the literature, the diagnosis of SBA is late because the symptoms can mimic a flare-up of IBD and the histological diagnosis is made after surgery. In our case, however, ultrasound enabled a timely diagnosis (only 2 weeks after symptom onset), and the ultrasound-guided percutaneous biopsy allowed for a histological diagnosis prior to surgery.

Below we present ultrasound images of further cases of intestinal cancers.

Case 2 Gastric adenocarcinoma in a 62-year-old woman with Crohn's disease on long term therapy with azathioprine; Presented with a three-month history of epigastralgia, weight loss, and sarcophobia (Figs. 11.21 and 11.22).

Case 3 Duodenal adenocarcinoma (Fig. 11.23) in a 45-year-old man with celiac disease and ulcerative colitis, poorly compliant with a gluten-free diet.

Case 4 Gastric linitis plastica in an 85-year-old female patient with Crohn's disease in poor general condition due to other comorbidities, bedridden for 1 year due to polyarthropathy; the patient complained of recurrent vomiting in the previous 6 months and a 15 kg weight loss (Fig. 11.24).

Case 5 Jejunal lymphoma in a 50-year-old overweight man with Crohn's disease; he complained of migrating abdominal pain for 2 months with associated sensation of heaviness (Figs. 11.25 and 11.26).

Case 6 Cecum cancer in a 70-year-old man with ulcerative colitis who had been suffering from pain in the right iliac fossa for 3 months with sudden onset of constipation and iron deficiency anemia, went to the emergency room for a subocclusive episode (Figs. 11.27, 11.28, and 11.29).

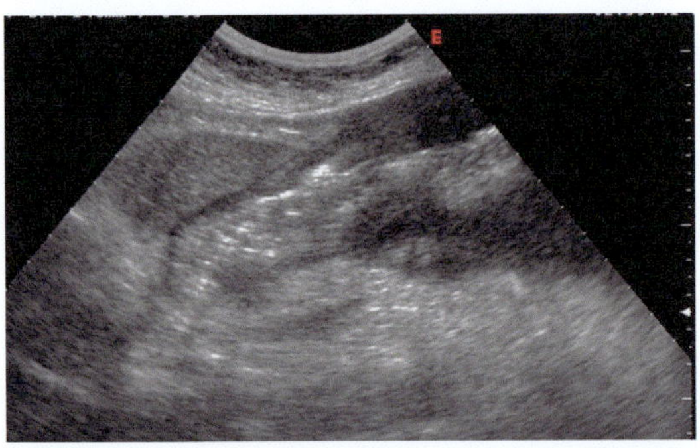

Fig. 11.21 Gastric antral wall thickening on ultrasound

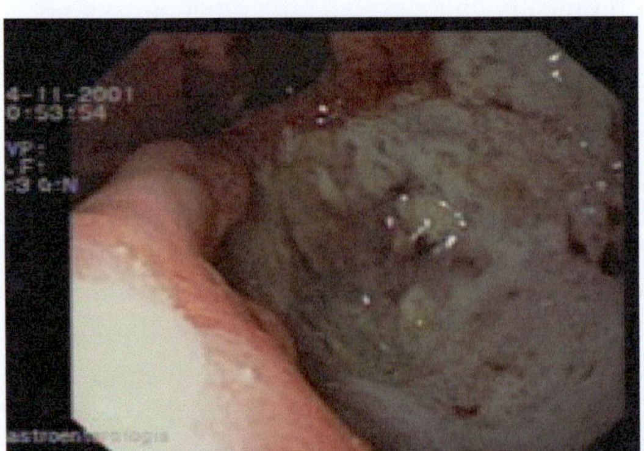

Fig. 11.22 On gastroscopy raised lesion with irregular margins, covered by a whitish plaque; biopsy revealed adenocarcinoma

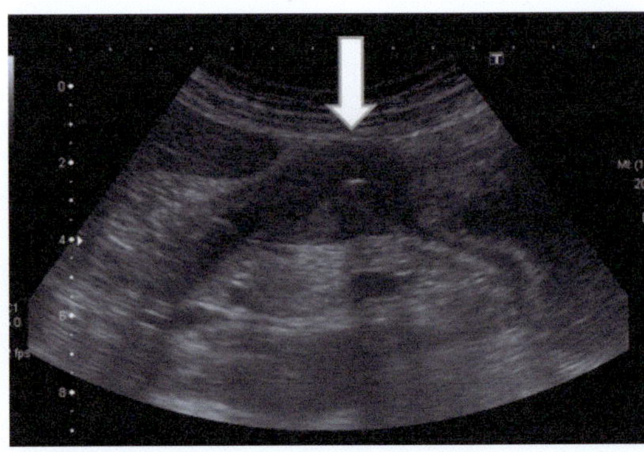

Fig. 11.23 Ultrasound shows hyperechoic lumen with hypoechoic wall with lost stratification in the initial loop of the duodenum

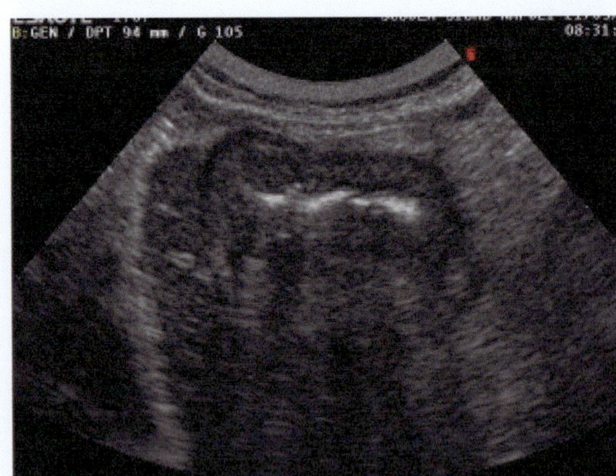

Fig. 11.24 Ultrasound

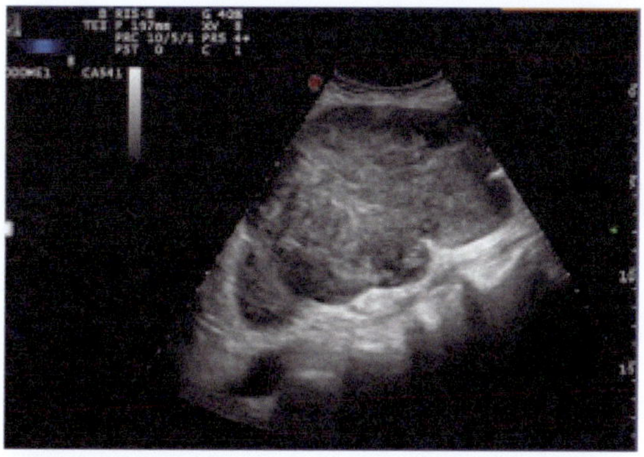

Fig. 11.25 Large, hypoechoic and heterogeneus mass in jejunum, difficult to identify lumen on ultrasound

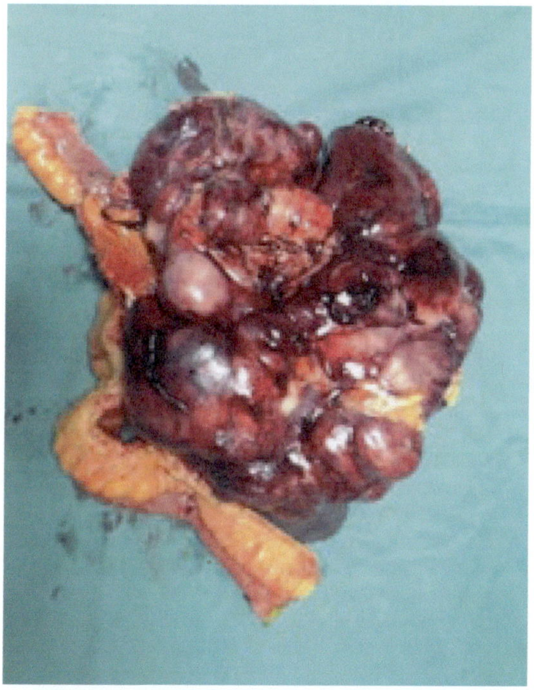

Fig. 11.26 Mass after removal

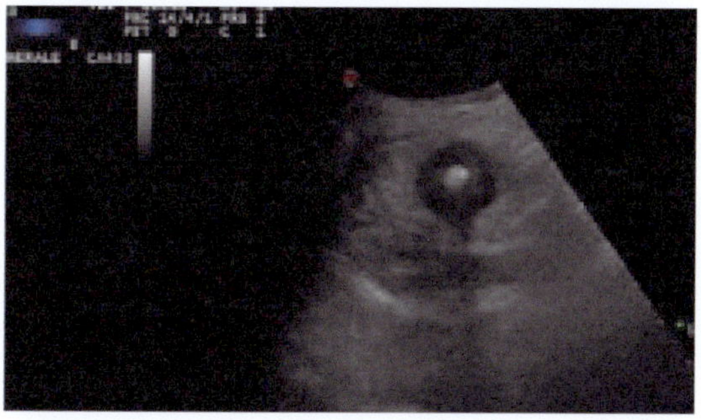

Fig. 11.27 Transverse scan of hypoechoic thickening of the cecal wall with marked hypertrophy of the surrounding mesentery

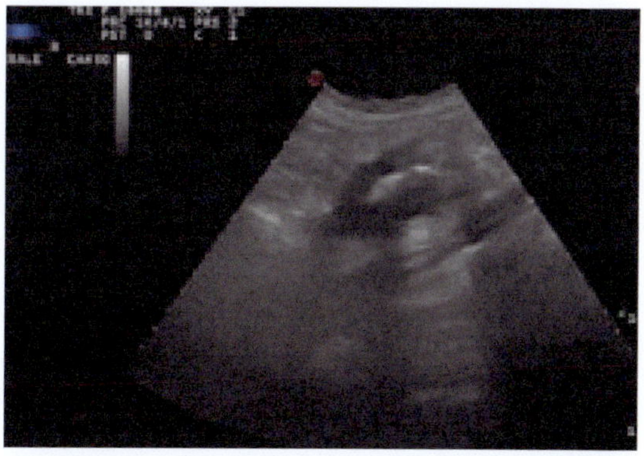

Fig. 11.28 Longitudinal scan

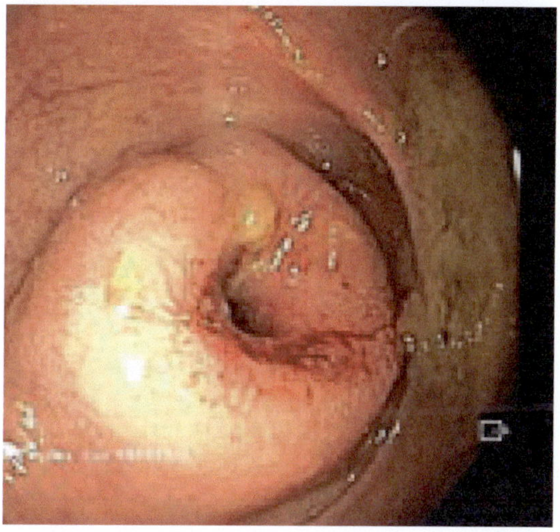

Fig. 11.29 Colonoscopy

Case 7 Gastric adenocarcinoma in a 57-year-old woman with ulcerative colitis with onset of epigastralgia, recurrent vomiting, anemia (Hb 7.5 g/dL), and weight loss of 8 kg since 1 month. At the initial gastroscopy, hypertrophy of the folds with unremarkable histology was documented (Fig. 11.30). On ultrasound examinations, marked and irregular thickening of the gastric body and fundus (Fig. 11.31) and intra- and perilesional vascular signals (Fig. 11.32) were detected, and a percutaneous ultrasound-guided biopsy allowed us to diagnose a gastric infiltrating adenocarcinoma.

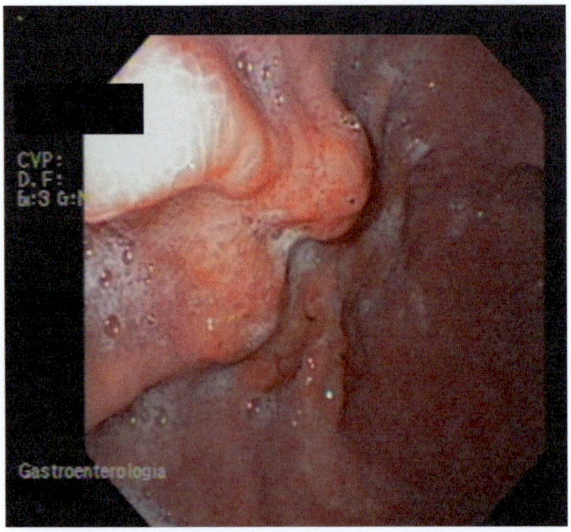

Fig. 11.30 Hypertrophy of the folds on gastroscopy

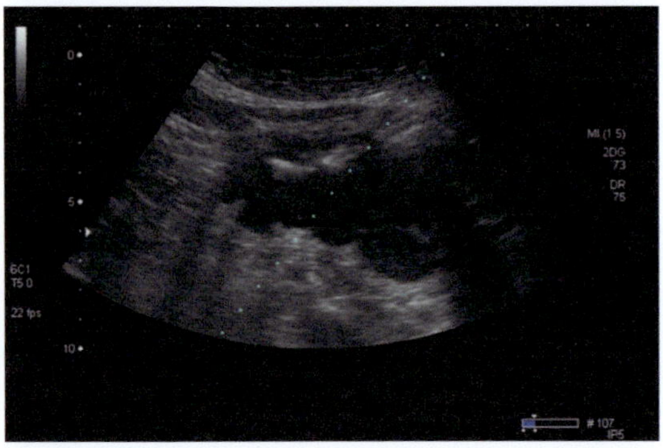

Fig. 11.31 Irregular thickening of the gastric body and fundus with discentric lumen

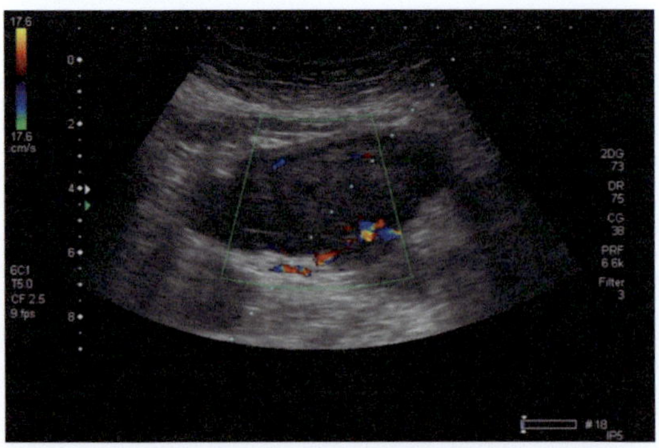

Fig. 11.32 Ultrasound with color Doppler

References

1. Edited, with an Introduction and Notes by Remer TG, Preface by Lewis WS. Serendipity and the three princes, from the Peregrinaggio of 1557. University of Oklahoma Press; 1965. LCC 65–10112.
2. Bor R, Fábián A, Szepes Z. Role of ultrasound in colorectal diseases. World J Gastroenterol. 2016;22(43):9477–87. https://doi.org/10.3748/wjg.v22.i43.9477. PMID: 27920469; PMCID: PMC5116592.
3. Terracciano F, Scalisi G, Attino V, Biscaglia G. A rare case of sigmoid colon obstruction in patient with ulcerative colitis: role of transabdominal ultrasound-guided biopsy. J Ultrasound. 2014;18(4):411–4. https://doi.org/10.1007/s40477-014-0105-6. Published 2014 Jun 13.
4. Shin LK, Halpern D, Weston SR, Meiner EM, Katz DS. Prospective CT diagnosis of stump appendicitis. AJR Am J Roentgenol. 2005;184:S62–4. https://doi.org/10.2214/ajr.184.3_supplement.01840s62.
5. Mangi AA, Berger DL. Stump appendicitis. Am Surg. 2000;66:739–41.
6. Walsh DC, Roediger WE. Stump appendicitis–a potential problem after laparoscopic appendicectomy. Surg Laparosc Endosc. 1997;7:357–8.
7. Dockerty MB, et al. A clinicopathologic study of the epiploic appendages. Surg Gynecol Obstet. 1956;103(4):423–33.
8. Rioux M, Langis P. Primary epiploic appendagitis: clinical, US, and CT findings in 14 cases. Radiology. 1994;191(2):523–6. https://doi.org/10.1148/radiology.191.2.8153333.
9. Desai HP, et al. Infarction of an epiploic appendage. Review of the literature. J Clin Gastroenterol. 1993;16(4):323–5. https://doi.org/10.1097/00004836-199306000-00012.
10. Haselkorn T, Whittemore AS, Lilienfeld DE. Incidence of small bowel cancer in the United States and worldwide: geographic, temporal, and racial differences. Cancer Causes Control. 2005;16:781–7. https://doi.org/10.1007/s10552-005-3635-6.
11. Bhatt H, Mathis KL. Small Bowel carcinoma in the setting of inflammatory Bowel disease. Clin Colon Rectal Surg. 2023;37(1):46–52. https://doi.org/10.1055/s-0043-1762929.
12. Dabaja BS, Suki D, Pro B, Bonnen M, Ajani J. Adenocarcinoma of the small bowel: presentation, prognostic factors, and outcome of 217 patients. Cancer. 2004;101:518–26. https://doi.org/10.1002/cncr.20404.
13. Kappelman MD, Farkas DK, Long MD, et al. Risk of cancer in patients with inflammatory bowel diseases: a nationwide population-based cohort study with 30 years of follow-up evaluation. Clin Gastroenterol Hepatol. 2014;12(02):265–730. https://doi.org/10.1016/j.cgh.2013.03.034.

MIX
Papier aus verantwortungsvollen Quellen
Paper from responsible sources
FSC® C105338

If you have any concerns about our products,
you can contact us on
ProductSafety@springernature.com

In case Publisher is established outside the EU,
the EU authorized representative is:
Springer Nature Customer Service Center GmbH
Europaplatz 3, 69115 Heidelberg, Germany

Printed by Libri Plureos GmbH
in Hamburg, Germany